Overcoming Postnatal Depression

A Five Areas Approach

Overcoming Postnatal Depression

A Five Areas Approach

Dr Chris Williams MBChB BSc MMedSc MD
FRCPsych BABCP accredited CBT practitioner, Registered
CBT therapist with UKCP
Senior Lecturer and Honorary Consultant
Psychiatrist, Section of Psychological Medicine,
Faculty of Medicine, University of Glasgow, UK

Dr Roch Cantwell MBChB BAO FRCPsych
Consultant Perinatal Psychiarist, NHS Greater
Glasgow and Clyde, and Honorary Senior
Lecturer, University of Glasgow, UK

Karen Robertson RMN, BSc PGDip in Cognitive
Behaviour Therapy
Associate Director of Nursing in Mental Health
and Learning Disability, NHS Lanarkshire, and
formerly Nurse Consultant, Perinatal Mental
Health, Perinatal Mental Health Service,
Southern General Hospital, Glasgow, UK

Helping you to help yourself
www.livinglifetothefull.com
www.fiveareas.com

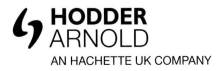

AN HACHETTE UK COMPANY

First published in Great Britain in 2009 by
Hodder Arnold, an imprint of Hodder Education
An Hachette UK Company, 338 Euston Road, London NW1 3BH

http://www.hoddereducation.com

Hachette's policy is to use papers that are natural, renewable and
recyclable products and made from wood grown in sustainable forests.
The logging and manufacturing processes are expected to conform to the
environmental regulations of the country of origin.

Whilst the advice and information in this book are believed to be true and
accurate at the date of going to press, neither the authors nor the
publisher can accept any legal responsibility or liability for any errors or
omissions that may be made.

British Library Cataloguing in Publication Data
A catalogue record for this book is available from the British Library

Library of Congress Cataloging-in-Publication Data
A catalog record for this book is available from the Library of Congress

ISBN-13 978-0-340-97234-2

2 3 4 5 6 7 8 9 10

Commissioning Editor: Philip Shaw
Project Editor: Amy Mulick
Production Controller: Karen Tate
Cover Design: Laura De Grasse

Typeset in 11/14pt Frutiger Light by Pantek Arts Ltd., Maidstone, Kent
Printed and bound in Malta

What do you think about this book? Or any other Hodder Arnold title?
Please visit our website: **www.hoddereducation.com** or send
comments to **admin@fiveareas.com**.

New ways of accessing the workbooks

 PDF versions of the workbooks are available from the publisher for restricted access on password-protected health service computer servers to allow high quality copies of the workbooks to be printed off by a defined number of practitioners or patients.

Buying the books in bulk: Bulk copies of the book are available at discounted rates direct from the publisher. To take advantage of this please contact: Jane MacRae, Sales Development Manager, Hodder Education, 338 Euston Road, London NW1 3BH. Tel: +44 (0) 20 7873 6146; email: **jane.macrae@hodder.co.uk**

Contents

Introduction

Welcome to *Overcoming Postnatal Depression: A Five Areas Approach*. This book is designed to actively help you:

- Learn important information about how postnatal depression can affect your life.
- Work out why you are feeling as you do.
- Learn and practise some proven practical skills to help change how you feel.

The aim is that you should be able to make helpful changes to your life with these clearly described practical tools that you can use yourself.

Who are the workbooks for?

You may be using the workbooks for yourself, or perhaps you are a close friend or family member wanting to know more about postnatal depression. Many healthcare practitioners also use the workbooks in this series to support those they work with.

Self-help approaches can be used by people with problems ranging from mild distress through to more severe depression. The key thing is that you feel **able** to use the materials and **want** to use this approach.

The course involves **reading** the course workbooks and also **working** on problems by putting into practice the things you are learning. Picking the right time to do the course is important. For example, if your concentration, energy or motivation levels are far lower than usual, you may find it very hard to keep your mind on things or to make changes. Other approaches such as anti-depressants may be more appropriate first – allowing you to come back to use the workbooks at a time when you are able to get the most from them. If you find that you struggle to use the workbooks, or you feel worse as you work through them, please discuss this with your doctor or other healthcare practitioner. The course is not meant to replace getting the right level of support for more severe mental health problems.

Using the workbooks

There is no right or wrong way to use the workbooks. Many people find it most helpful to first read the two workbooks in Part 1 (*Starting out* and *Understanding why you feel as you do*) to help gain an overview of the approach. This will also help you to decide which of the *Making changes* workbooks in Part 2 of the book you should read. You can use as many or as few workbooks in the course as you wish. You will feel most motivated to try to make changes if you use the workbooks that tackle problems you have noticed in your life. The key to creating change in your life is **using** the workbooks and **putting what you learn into practice**.

Helping you stay on track

You may have found out about these workbooks in different ways. Sometimes a health practitioner will recommend them to help you tackle problems such as low mood or distress. Health practitioners can really help keep you on track and stay motivated in putting what you have learned into practice. Recent research has also shown that this sort of support and encouragement from a practitioner or other supporter can make a really big difference in how much people recover and how much they get out of books like this. We therefore strongly suggest that you work through these resources with support and encouragement from a practitioner or support worker, or someone else such as a voluntary sector worker. They can help guide you and encourage you to put what you are learning into practice.

Getting the most from your support

If you are receiving support from a practitioner, part of the trick to getting the most from the course is having a plan. Work together to plan what you are going to work on – and when you will do it. Many people find it helpful to create an agenda of things to cover when you discuss your progress with your practitioner. An agenda to help you plan this meeting in order to get the most from it is included on page 18, and is freely available online at **www.fiveareas.com**.

Getting help from others

Sometimes people prefer to largely work on things by themselves. Even so, we suggest that you let your own doctor know you are using these workbooks, and you may find others, such as families and friends (see *Information for families and friends – how can you offer the best support?*), can be a real help. The key is knowing when to seek help from others if you are struggling.

A word of encouragement

Depression in the weeks and months after giving birth is common. Fortunately, it has now become clear that by changing certain thoughts and behaviour patterns you can greatly improve how you feel. The content of these workbooks is based on the cognitive behaviour therapy (CBT; a kind of talking treatment) approach. The developers of CBT have found many effective ways of tackling the common symptoms and problems faced when you feel low. This course is written in a way that explains what to do clearly so that you can test the effect of these different suggestions in your own life. The workbooks aim to help you to **regain a sense of control** over how you feel.

Sometimes making changes is easier said (or written) than done. All of us feel discouraged and overwhelmed from time to time. This is even more likely to occur in times of low mood. Therefore, **we would like to encourage you to try to make a commitment to use this course** and to keep at it even if you feel discouraged or stuck for a time. To do this you will need to **pace yourself** by using a step-by-step approach. Having someone else to encourage you is also important. The research on these approaches shows just how helpful this can be. Also, be realistic. Bear in mind what your motivation and energy levels allow you to do so you don't bite off more than you can chew. This will help you to get as much from the course as you can at the moment.

The *Starting out* workbook gives some suggestions of how you can **pace things**, and also some suggestions of what to do if you are struggling.

New online resources

Two online resources are available to support users of the course:

- **www.livinglifetothefull.com**. This completely free website contains short talks that help you to build upon the course workbooks. There is also a moderated discussion forum where people can swap ideas, hints and tips, as well as offering and receiving mutual support. Recent research strongly suggests that this site is a helpful treatment for depression.
- The **www.fiveareas.com** website points to other Five Areas resources including self-help books, free handouts and downloads (including MP3s of relaxation techniques) and more.

A note about copyright

This book once purchased in book form may be copied by the user as many times as required for use by themselves, or (if a practitioner) in their own personal clinical practice or in training. The content may not be reproduced on websites or emailed to others without permission.

Acknowledgements

The illustrations in the workbooks have been produced by Keith Chan, kchan75@hotmail.com. Copies are available as a separate download for clinical use at www.fiveareas.com.

Finally, we wish to thank Alison, Hannah, Andrew, Miriam and Brian who have supported us during the writing of this book

Dr Chris Williams, Dr Roch Cantwell, Karen Robertson
October 2008

PART 1

Understanding why you feel as you do

Overcoming Postnatal Depression
A Five Areas Approach

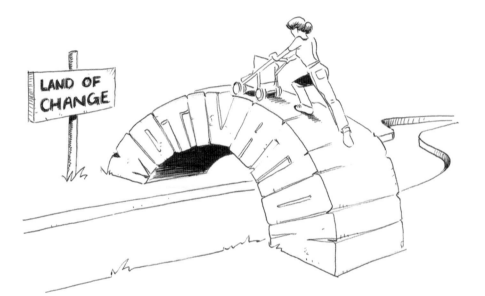

Starting out ... and how to keep going if you feel stuck

www.livinglifetothefull.com
www.fiveareas.com

Dr Chris Williams, Dr Roch Cantwell and
Karen Robertson

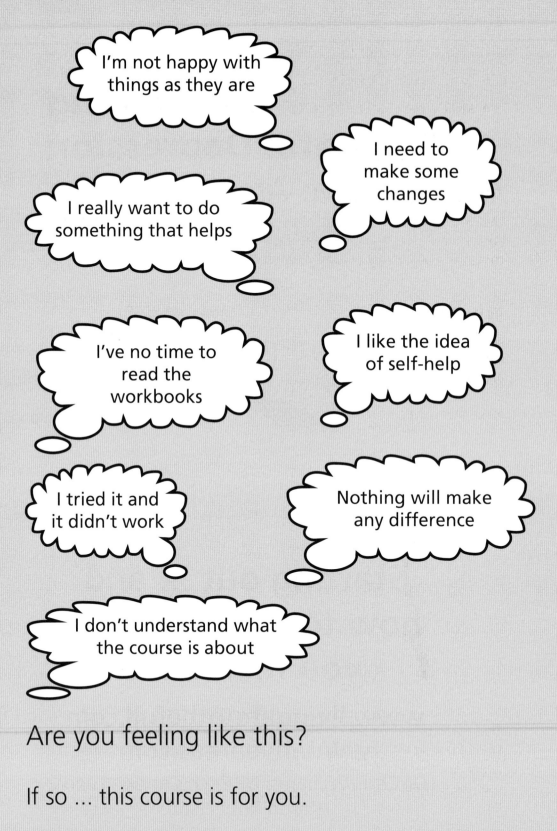

Are you feeling like this?

If so … this course is for you.

> # In this course you will:
>
> - Learn how to get the most out of this course.
> - Make a clear but flexible plan of when to use the workbooks.
> - Discover how to overcome common blocks to change.

About the course

The workbooks in this course aim to help you understand why you feel as you do. They will teach you important life skills that will help you to turn the corner, and tackle your postnatal depression.

Why should you use these workbooks?

Often people use these workbooks because they want to find out more about why they feel as they do, and also how to make changes. **You, the reader, are in control** – and you can work on things at a time that suits you. Time and time again people are surprised to see the amount of change they can make themselves using a self-help approach.

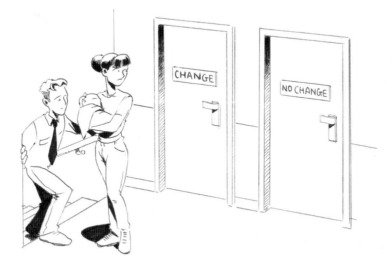

These workbooks use an approach called cognitive behaviour therapy (CBT, a kind of talking treatment). Don't worry though – there won't be any more jargon like that in the rest of the course. But you need to know that the course uses the CBT approach. Lots of research has proved that self-help materials based on the CBT approach work well for problems such as depression and anxiety. And CBT self-help is recommended for use in the National Health Service (NHS) in the UK as a treatment for mild to moderate depression. Research on one of the other books in this series has also confirmed the effectiveness as a treatment for depression.

In this course, each workbook will teach you how to make changes in different areas of your life in clear, step-by-step ways.

Getting going

Well done! You've done something that quite a few people struggle to do – **you are still reading**.

It can sometimes seem really hard starting to change. Have you ever bought or been given a book or a DVD and never even opened it or taken the wrapper off? Using this course is no different. In fact, in some ways it's harder because it's not a book that's there for entertainment. Instead these are **work**books – which aim to enable you to change how you feel.

What should I read first?

You usually start the course by working through these two workbooks:

- This one – *Starting out*.

- And then *Understanding why you feel as you do*.

The *Understanding why you feel as you do* workbook will help you to start working out how postnatal depression is affecting you. It will also help you decide which other workbooks you wish to work on.

Key point

Choose the workbooks **you** want to work on – making sure they deal with the problems/difficulties **you** are facing.

Developing a routine

Have you ever noticed how our surroundings can affect how we feel? For example, if you are used to having a snack while you watch television, sometimes just sitting in the same chair can make you feel hungry!

In the same way you might wish to set aside a particular place to complete the workbooks. For example, sitting on a chair at the kitchen table (your 'workbook chair') with a pen and some blank paper to jot down ideas as you read. It also makes sense to try to plan enough time so that you can get really involved in the workbook – preferably half an hour or so, if you feel you have sufficient energy and concentration for this.

Planning how and when to use the workbooks

It is often helpful to actively plan completing the workbooks into your day and diary rather than just 'trying to fit it in some time'. The best plans say:

- **What** you are going to do.

- **When** you are going to do it.

and

- **Predict** things that might block or get in the way of you doing this.

You may find the following **Planning task** helpful in making this regular commitment. Please use it to help plan how to use the next key workbook: *Understanding why you feel as you do*. This workbook will help you decide which other course workbooks you might need to use.

Your plan to use the workbooks

 Task

 When are you going to read the *Understanding why you feel as you do* workbook?

Write the day and time when you plan to do this here:

Is reading some of it every day practical for you? If not every day, is every other day more realistic? Many people with low mood notice they feel at their worst first thing in the morning. So you might find that the best time for you to read the workbooks is after lunch, in the late afternoon or in the early evening. Think about what you know of your baby's routine or you could pick a time when others are around to help look after your baby.

Q **How much will you read at a time?**

Write down your plan of how much you will read here:

Many people find it easier to read just a few pages at a time – making sure that you stop, think and reflect by answering the questions as you do this.

Q **Is this realistic, practical and achievable?**

You know your own life and its various demands and commitments. In particular, you know your baby and other demands on your life.

Q **What problems could block or prevent you doing this, and how can you overcome these?**

For example, what if your baby cries, wakes up or needs a nappy change. Write your possible blocks in here:

Q How could you unblock them?

Getting into the mood: doing something physical can help you get started

You are likely to feel physically and mentally sluggish when you feel low or when you aren't sleeping well. You may be doing very little during the day and it may be hard to see yourself making any changes.

A good start to using the workbooks is to do something physical first. For example, get up and walk around the room and – if you have them – up and down the stairs. Then sit down on your 'workbook chair' – such as an upright kitchen chair that forces you to sit up rather than slump back. Now start reading the workbook.

But what about the baby?

All this sounds very straightforward, doesn't it? Sitting down and planning a time to work. But having a baby makes planning anything very difficult. Things will slowly become easier, as your baby settles into his or her own routine. But to begin with, it might well be a case of taking the time when you can. As your baby gets older, he or she will probably sleep at more predictable times – for example after feeds, or in the afternoon. Or perhaps sometimes someone else can come round and help out while you work on things.

Here are some suggestions of how to build on this first step during the rest of the course.

Some dos and don'ts for getting the most out of the course
Do:

- Try and work through one workbook a week.

- **Get a pen.** Writing things down means you are thinking and learning. In fact it's more than that. Sometimes **you actually work out what you really think** about something when you speak it out loud or write it down.

- Answer all the questions – and really try to stop, think and reflect as you read.

- Ask: How does this apply to me? How might I use this in my life?

- Try out what you read in the workbooks. A specific section at the end of each workbook will help you to decide how to do this. Have you any ideas so far? Take what helps and use it again and again.

- Be realistic. You are more likely to succeed if you try changing things one step at a time rather than throwing yourself into things and then running out of steam.

- Make notes in the **My notes** section at the end of each workbook. Also re-read sections of the workbooks and your notes to go over what you have learned. It may be that different parts become clearer, or seem more useful on second reading.

- Use the workbooks to build up the help you receive in other ways, such as talking to friends, or from self-help organisations and support groups.

Don't:

- Expect a sudden miracle cure. Change takes time and practice.

- Try to do this completely on your own. Supportive encouragement from a trusted friend, health visitor or another health professional can really help.

- Try to read the workbook against the odds, such as times when you are trying to soothe your baby.

- Cut yourself off from other useful supports. You can do this course alongside other treatments, such as seeing a health worker or taking an anti-depressant. These approaches can all be helpful parts of moving forwards.

Helping you stay on track

You may have found out about these workbooks in different ways. Sometimes a health practitioner will recommend them to help you tackle problems such as low mood or distress. Health practitioners can really help keep you on track and stay motivated in putting what you have learned into practice. Recent research has also shown that this sort of support and encouragement from a practitioner or other supporter can make a really big difference in how much people recover and how much they get out of books like this. We therefore strongly suggest that you work through these resources with support and encouragement from a practitioner or support worker, or someone else such as a voluntary sector worker. They can help guide you and encourage you to put what you are learning into practice.

Getting the most from your support

If you are receiving support from a practitioner, part of the trick to getting the most from the course is having a plan. Work together to plan what you are going to work on – and when you will do it. Many people find it helpful to create an agenda of things to cover when you discuss your progress with your practitioner. An agenda to help you plan this meeting in order to get the most from it is included at the end of this workbook, and is freely available online at **www.fiveareas.com**.

Getting help from others

Sometimes people prefer to largely work on things by themselves. Even so, we suggest that you let your own doctor know you are using these workbooks, and you may find others, such as families and friends (see *Information for families and friends – how can you offer the best support?*), can be a real help. The key is knowing when to seek help from others if you are struggling.

Finding extra support

Having someone around who can offer *support and encouragement* can help. This is especially important if you feel you are struggling or feel stuck. Sometimes just the act of telling someone – a family member, friend or health worker – that you are working on something, or plan to do a certain activity on a particular day, can really help. Just knowing that someone else may ask you how it's going could help spur you into action. You might go through your answers to the questions in the workbooks with them – or keep your answers private and only discuss some of the course content.

That could even ask them to do the workbook that's specially for them. (*Information for families and friends – how can you offer the best support?*). That workbook aims to help them understand how best to support and encourage you.

Building your motivation to change

Motivation is usually low during times of depression. You may be sleeping poorly, have low energy levels and struggle to be motivated to change.

It might help if you write yourself the following **letter**. Try to do this now, before moving on, even if it seems hard to do.

Imagine it is 10 years in the future. You have made important changes in your life and things are much better. You have achieved many of the goals you have set yourself. Write yourself an **encouraging letter** about why you need to make changes now.

Dear (your name)

Signed:

(Myself)

Change takes time

Sometimes it's easy to forget how hard it is to learn new information or skills that you now take for granted. Think about some of the skills you have learned over the years. For example, if you can drive or swim or ride a bike, think back to your first driving/swimming lesson or attempt to cycle without stabilisers. You probably weren't very good at it that first time, yet with practice you developed the skills needed to do it. In the same way, you can overcome low mood and tension by practising what you learn – even if it may seem hard at first.

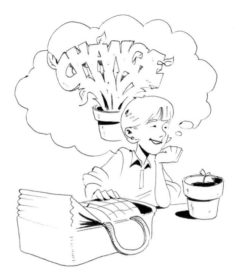

Write down some other things you have learnt that took time:

Key point

You can't expect to be able to swim immediately. You may need to start at the shallow end and practise at first. Use the workbooks in a similar way. Pace what you do and don't jump immediately and enthusiastically into the deep end.

Having realistic expectations

It's important not to approach this course either far too positively or far too negatively. It would be untrue to claim that if you use this course you are guaranteed results. What we can guarantee is that this approach has helped many thousands of people – and that the workbooks teach clinically proved approaches that have been a help for many. Hopefully, at the very least you will learn some interesting and helpful things along the way.

Common problems in using the course

I've no time

Having a baby means that time is always going to be short. There will be many demands on your time. But …

Task

Imagine you have a close friend who has postnatal depression. She doesn't like how she feels – and you know that it is affecting her in lots of different ways. What helpful advice would you give her if she said 'I don't have time'.

Write down your encouraging advice here:

… if you would give your friend this advice to make some time, could you use that same advice yourself?

I feel too down to do this now

Sometimes in severe postnatal depression, it might not be the right time to use these workbooks. But you can always come back to them later if you are finding that things are too much now. If you can't concentrate for long just go at a pace you can manage. You should also discuss your treatment options with your doctor.

I'll never change

One big block to getting better is not believing that you can change. Many people find that they gain much more from the course than they first thought they would. Could this be true for you?

Again, imagine if your friend told you she believed she would never change from a time of low mood. She needs encouragement.

📌 Task

What words of encouragement would you say to her? Write them down here:

If you would offer helpful and positive advice to a friend, then why not also offer it to yourself?

Experiment

Even if you have doubts about the course, or about your ability to use it effectively, try to give it a go. In this way you can test it out in your own life. If you still find it doesn't help after you've given it a good go that would be a sensible time to try something different.

Summary

Well done – you've got to the last section and you're still reading! That's a very important achievement. So many people who want to change find it hard starting out.

Let's review what you have learned in this workbook. You have covered:

- How to get the most out of the course.

- How to write a clear but flexible plan of when to use the workbooks.

- How to overcome common blocks to change.

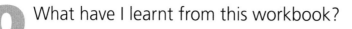

Q What have I learnt from this workbook?

Q What do I want to try *next*?

Putting into practice what you have learned

You are likely to make the most progress if you can put into practice what you have learned in the workbook. Each workbook will encourage you to do this by suggesting certain tasks for you to do in the following days.

Suggested practice plan

Read the *Understanding why you feel as you do* workbook next. Use the **Planning task** on pages 7–9 to plan this. This workbook will help you work out which other course workbooks are relevant to you.

Other sources of support

 www.livinglifetothefull.com

This popular resource is designed to support readers of this workbook. This website is run by Dr Chris Williams, and is supported by NHS Greater Glasgow and Clyde, but is freely accessible to anyone, wherever they live. Many other supports are also available for people with low mood and depression. These are listed on the Living Life to the Full website.

 www.fiveareas.com

This website provides access to other Five Areas books and resources, including free handouts and resources such as relaxation MP3 files.

A request for feedback

An important part in the development of all the Five Areas assessment workbooks is that the content is updated on a regular basis, based on feedback from users and practitioners. If there are areas in this course that you find hard to understand, or seemed poorly written, please let us know (see contact details below). However, we can't answer specific questions or provide advice on treatment.

Address: Five Areas, PO Box 9, Glasgow G63 0WL, UK

 Our website: **www.fiveareas.com**
email: **feedback@fiveareas.com**

Acknowledgments

The cartoon illustrations in the workbooks have been produced by Keith Chan, kchan75@hotmail.com.

My Agenda for my next support session

If you are working with a support worker/practitioner, this agenda can help you plan to get the most from your sessions with them.

My review day:

Date:

Since my last review:

What's gone well?

What hasn't gone so well?

What have I learned from this?

My Progress Review

My Notes

Which workbook will I do next?:

Other tasks to take things forwards

1. What am I going to do?

2. When am I going to do it?

Is my planned task one that:

Q   Will be useful for understanding or changing how I am?
Yes ☐   No ☐

Q   Is a specific task so that I will know when I have done it?
Yes ☐   No ☐

Q   Is realistic: is it practical and achievable?   Yes ☐   No ☐

3. What problems/difficulties could arise, and how can I overcome them?

My next support session* (time/date) _____

*Remember to re-arrange this if you can't make the session

PLEASE NOTE: If you are struggling or feel worse, or if at any time you feel suicidal, please visit your doctor, go to A+E or phone NHS Direct (England and Wales) or NHS 24 (Scotland).

Overcoming Postnatal Depression

A Five Areas Approach

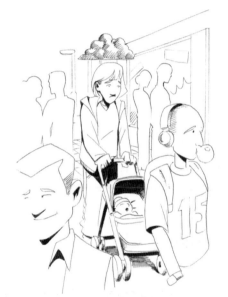

Understanding why you feel as you do

www.livinglifetothefull.com
www.fiveareas.com

Dr Chris Williams, Dr Roch Cantwell and Karen Robertson

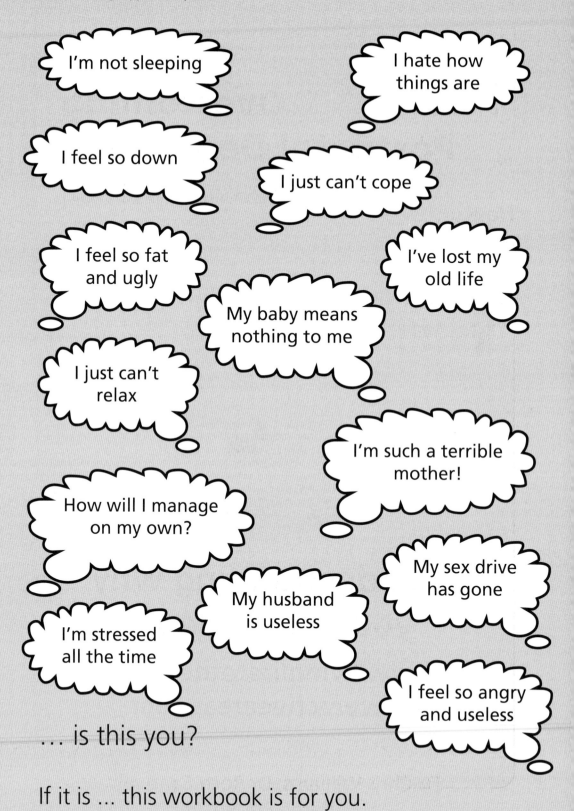

... is this you?

If it is ... this workbook is for you.

This workbook will help you to:

● Find out why you are feeling low, stressed and upset.

● Make some step-by-step changes so that you begin to feel better.

The first step to feeling good is working out why you are feeling bad.

How did things get to be like this?

Anyone can feel depressed and stressed if their emotional balance is upset. You can use a time line to find out how you started to feel this way. An example is shown below.

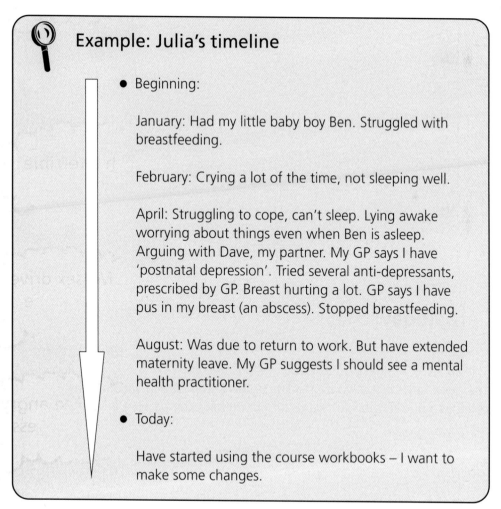

Example: Julia's timeline

● Beginning:

January: Had my little baby boy Ben. Struggled with breastfeeding.

February: Crying a lot of the time, not sleeping well.

April: Struggling to cope, can't sleep. Lying awake worrying about things even when Ben is asleep. Arguing with Dave, my partner. My GP says I have 'postnatal depression'. Tried several anti-depressants, prescribed by GP. Breast hurting a lot. GP says I have pus in my breast (an abscess). Stopped breastfeeding.

August: Was due to return to work. But have extended maternity leave. My GP suggests I should see a mental health practitioner.

● Today:

Have started using the course workbooks – I want to make some changes.

Task

Now it's your turn. Fill in your own time line below.

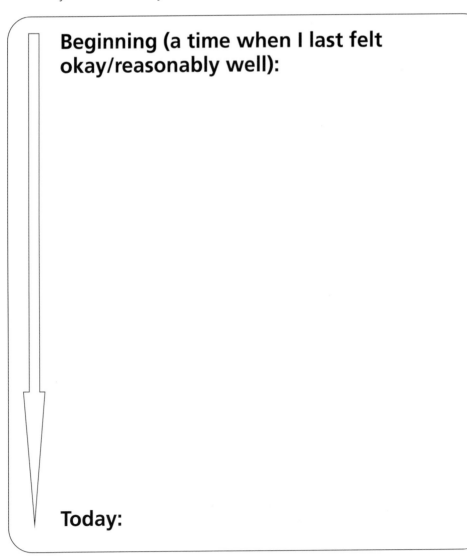

Beginning (a time when I last felt okay/reasonably well):

Today:

The good news is that your time line doesn't stop here. If you can make changes, you can move forwards and bring back the balance in your life.

Feeling out of balance – when things feel worse and worse

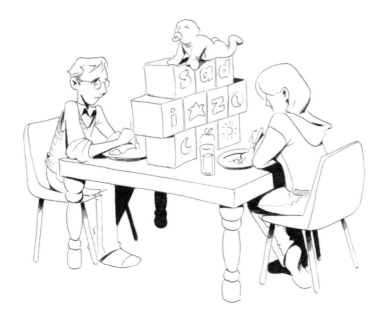

Normally, most people feel **able to cope** with the problems they face. When you are in balance, you know you can deal with your problems. So it isn't your situation or problem alone that causes you to feel down or stressed. Instead it's how you think about these things that makes you feel like you do. And dwelling on problems and getting things out of perspective doesn't help you feel better or make your problems go away.

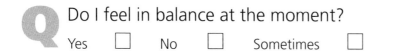

Q Do I feel in balance at the moment?

Yes ☐   No ☐   Sometimes ☐

If you feel out of balance some or all of the time, this course can help you get your balance back.

Let's start by finding out more about the Five Areas Approach. This Approach can help you understand how your lowered mood affects your life.

Understanding how you feel using the Five Areas Approach

One helpful way of understanding how low mood and depression affects you is to think of the ways that they can affect the different areas of your life. The **Five Areas Approach** can help you to do this by looking in detail at five important areas of your life.

The Five Areas are:

- Area 1: Your situation. This includes the **people and events around you**.

- Area 2: Your **thinking**. This can often become extreme and unhelpful when you feel low.

- Area 3: Your **feelings** (also called moods or emotions).

- Area 4: Any **altered physical symptoms** in your body.

- Area 5: Your **altered behaviour or activity levels**. This includes both the helpful things you do, which make you feel better, and the unhelpful things you do, which backfire and make you feel even worse.

Try to think about how the Five Areas assessment can help Julia understand how she is feeling.

Example: How postnatal depression is affecting Julia's life

Julia had her son Ben in January. At first things went well although breastfeeding was a struggle. Over the next few weeks Julia felt more and more tired. She found it hard to sleep or even relax – even when Ben was asleep. She felt exhausted and tearful over things she would normally cope with.

By April Julia felt she was failing in everything. She was struggling to cope, couldn't sleep and was lying awake, beating herself up that she was using formula milk. She had started giving Ben formula milk after she had a breast abscess and found breastfeeding too sore. Julia felt her partner Dave wasn't helping enough and this led to many arguments and critical words.

By August Julia realised she couldn't cope with returning to work and informed her manager that she was going to take the full year's maternity leave. But this only made her sense of failing at things worse. She sits on a different chair from Dave every evening, and they have stopped having sex and cuddles. Julia also prefers to stay in and has started to isolate herself from her family and friends. She dwells on thoughts that she is a bad mother and then gets upset because she feels nothing for Ben except anger and resentment. This makes her feel even more guilty as she knows she should love him.

The figure below shows how Julia's problems can be summarised using the Five Areas Approach.

Julia's Five Areas summary

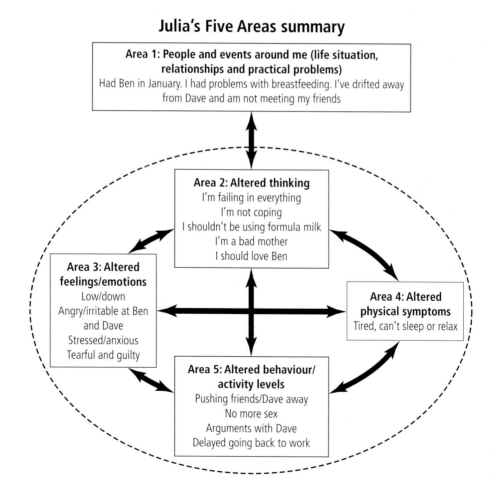

Area 1: People and events around me (life situation, relationships and practical problems)
Had Ben in January. I had problems with breastfeeding. I've drifted away from Dave and am not meeting my friends

Area 2: Altered thinking
I'm failing in everything
I'm not coping
I shouldn't be using formula milk
I'm a bad mother
I should love Ben

Area 3: Altered feelings/emotions
Low/down
Angry/irritable at Ben and Dave
Stressed/anxious
Tearful and guilty

Area 4: Altered physical symptoms
Tired, can't sleep or relax

Area 5: Altered behaviour/ activity levels
Pushing friends/Dave away
No more sex
Arguments with Dave
Delayed going back to work

The Five Areas diagram shows that what you think about a situation or problem can affect how you feel physically and emotionally. It also shows that your thinking affects what you do (your behaviour or activity levels). Look at the arrows in the diagram. Each of the Five Areas of your life (your situation, your relationships or practical problems, your thinking, your emotional and physical feelings, and your behaviour changes) affect each other.

📌 Task

Can the Five Areas Approach help you understand why you feel as you do? Take a look at what's happening for you in each of the Five Areas, starting with Area 1.

Area 1: People and events around you

All of us from time to time face practical problems such as:

- Problems with family and life at home.
- The challenges of a new baby or bringing up young children.
- Problems in relationships with partners or friends or colleagues.
- Other life challenges, for example returning to work, college, etc.

People who have had a relationship split, or who have no-one to talk to, can also get depression. Mothers facing the demands of trying to bring up young children are also at greater risk of depression. Low mood and tension can affect any kind of relationship. You may become confused about your feelings towards others, and you can lose interest in your relationships. Love can feel subdued. For example, a new mother may look at her baby and feel nothing – this is a common symptom in postnatal depression. Similarly, those with a spiritual faith may feel they struggle to get the support that they usually get from their faith.

Are any of these relevant to you?

- There is no one around who I can really talk to.

  Yes ☐   No ☐   Sometimes ☐

- I am struggling to cope with my baby.

  Yes ☐   No ☐   Sometimes ☐

- My baby isn't feeding easily.

  Yes ☐   No ☐   Sometimes ☐

- My baby isn't sleeping well.

  Yes ☐   No ☐   Sometimes ☐

- My children won't do what I tell them.

  Yes ☐   No ☐   Sometimes ☐

- I worry about work or money or debts.

  Yes ☐   No ☐   Sometimes ☐

- There are problems where I live.

  Yes ☐   No ☐   Sometimes ☐

- It's hard to get on with another person/people in my family.

  Yes ☐   No ☐   Sometimes ☐

- I am having problems with my neighbours.

  Yes ☐   No ☐   Sometimes ☐

- I have problems with colleagues at work.

  Yes ☐   No ☐   Sometimes ☐

- My family has unemployment/job worries.

  Yes ☐   No ☐   Sometimes ☐

- My family has housing problems.

  Yes ☐   No ☐   Sometimes ☐

Task

Now write down any other problems you may have. You may also find it helpful to write in more detail about any of the problems you noted in the previous list. Use an extra sheet of paper if you need to, or use the **My Notes** section at the end of this workbook.

Summary for Area 1: People and events around you

After answering the questions, rate the extent of your problems in this area.

No problems at all   The worst they could possibly be

| 0 | 1 | 2 | 3 | 4 | 5 | 6 | 7 | 8 | 9 | 10 |

What next?

Looking at the graph, check whether the people and events around you (your situation) is an area you wish to work on. If you do, two of the workbooks in the course will help you to rebalance relationships (*Being assertive* and *Building relationships with your baby, family and friends*) and begin to tackle practical problems (*Practical problem solving*). You or your family or friends may also find some good ideas in the *Information for families and friends* workbook.

Do you need help from other people?

Sometimes your problems in your relationships or your situation are so difficult that you need help from others. If you or your baby/children are at risk of significant harm or abuse then you need to ask others for help. Your own GP (if you are not registered you can look for one at **www.yell.co.uk**), NHS Direct (tel **0845 4647**), NHS 24 (Scotland; tel **08454 24 24 24**) or your local hospital's emergency department can be helpful. Think of contacting a 24-hour helpline, such as the National Society for the Prevention of Cruelty to Children (NSPCC) helpline, if you think your child or children's welfare is at risk. You will find contact details for useful sources of help at the end of the workbook.

Area 2: Your thinking

When someone feels low, how they **think** tends to change. You tend to lose confidence and find it harder to make decisions. You may worry about things you have done – and things you haven't done. You begin to see everything in quite negative ways.

So your thinking becomes:

- Extreme.

- Unhelpful.

> ### Example: How you think can affect how you feel
>
> You are shopping in a supermarket when your daughter starts crying. Nothing you do helps. You give her a cuddle and try to distract her but she continues to shout and cry. As other shoppers go by you think 'She's doing this on purpose to embarrass me.' You blush and cringe with embarrassment and your body feels very tense. You start to feel really angry and shout at her to 'Just shut up and stop whining!.' You leave the shop and feel very embarrassed.
>
> But if the same situation occurred and you had thought 'She must be hungry' you would have felt and behaved differently.
>
> We can all fall into unhelpful patterns of thinking when we feel low or distressed.

Have you noticed any of these common unhelpful patterns of thinking in your life?

Unhelpful thinking pattern	Do you ever think this way? (Put a tick in the box if you have noticed this thinking style – even if it is just sometimes.) Write down an example
Being your own worst critic/bias against yourself For example, being very critical and biased against yourself; overlooking your strengths; seeing yourself as not coping; or not recognising your achievements	☐
Putting a negative slant on things (negative mental filter) For example, seeing things through dark-tinted glasses; seeing the glass as being half empty rather than half full; that whatever you do in the week it's never enough to give you a sense of achievement; tending to focus on the bad side of everyday situations	☐
Have a gloomy view of the future For example, thinking that things will stay bad or get even worse; predicting that things will go wrong; or always looking for the next thing to fail	☐
Jumping to the worst conclusion For example, predicting that the very worst outcome will happen, thinking that you will fail very badly	☐
Having a negative view about how others see you (mind-reading) For example, often thinking that others don't like you or think badly of you for no particular reason	☐

Unfairly taking responsibility for things ☐

For example, thinking you should take the blame if things go wrong; feeling guilty about things that are not really your fault; and thinking that you are responsible for everyone else

---

Making extreme statements/rules ☐

For example:

● Using the words '*always*', '*never*' a lot to summarise things.

● If a bad thing happens, saying '*Just typical*' because it seems this always happens.

● Making myself a lot of 'must', '*should*' '*ought*' or '*got to*' rules.

● Believing I must always push myself to do things well.

Summary for Area 2: Your thinking

After answering the questions, rate the extent of your problems in this area.

No problems at all   The worst they could possibly be

0	1	2	3	4	5	6	7	8	9	10

What next?

If this is an area you wish to work on, the *Noticing and changing extreme and unhelpful thinking* workbook will help you to find out and change these ways of thinking.

Area 3: Your feelings/emotions

Q Which emotional changes have you noticed over the past two weeks?

- Lowness or sadness.

  Yes ☐   No ☐   Sometimes ☐

- Reduced or no sense of pleasure in things.

  Yes ☐   No ☐   Sometimes ☐

- Loss of all feelings, for example noticing no feelings at all.

  Yes ☐   No ☐   Sometimes ☐

- Guilt.

  Yes ☐   No ☐   Sometimes ☐

- Worry, stress, tension, anxiety or panic.

  Yes ☐   No ☐   Sometimes ☐

- Anger or irritability.

  Yes ☐   No ☐   Sometimes ☐

- Shame or embarrassment.

  Yes ☐   No ☐   Sometimes ☐

- Other (write down here):

Your emotions are an important and normal part of your life. Changes in how you feel are often linked with your thoughts, memories and the ideas that are going through your mind at the time. Try to become aware of these thoughts and note them when there is a change in how you feel (your emotions).

The good news is that by noticing these changes you can begin to slowly make helpful changes in how you feel.

Summary for Area 3: Your feelings/emotions

After answering the questions, rate the extent of your problems in this area.

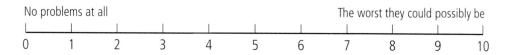

No problems at all   The worst they could possibly be

0   1   2   3   4   5   6   7   8   9   10

What next?

If this is an area you wish to work on then making helpful changes in any of the other four areas will lead to positive changes in how you feel emotionally.

Area 4: Your altered physical symptoms

Usually when people feel very low, they notice having physical symptoms at the same time.

Q Which physical symptoms have you noticed over the past two weeks?

- Are you waking up earlier than usual?

    Yes ☐   No ☐   Sometimes ☐

- Are you finding it hard getting off to sleep – even when your baby is settled?

    Yes ☐   No ☐   Sometimes ☐

- Are you waking up at night – even when your baby is settled?

    Yes ☐   No ☐   Sometimes ☐

- Has your appetite increased or decreased?

  Yes ☐   No ☐   Sometimes ☐

- Have you put on or lost weight?

  Yes ☐   No ☐   Sometimes ☐

- Do you feel as if you don't have enough energy to do things?

  Yes ☐   No ☐   Sometimes ☐

- Have you stopped having sex or aren't interested as much in it as before?

  Yes ☐   No ☐   Sometimes ☐

- Are you constipated?

  Yes ☐   No ☐   Sometimes ☐

- Do you feel any pain?

  Yes ☐   No ☐   Sometimes ☐

- Do you feel restless?

  Yes ☐   No ☐   Sometimes ☐

- Do you have any other symptoms?

Summary for Area 4: Your altered physical symptoms

Having answering the questions, rate the extent of your problems in this area.

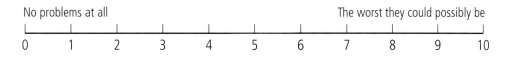

No problems at all									The worst they could possibly be
0	1	2	3	4	5	6	7	8	9	10

What next?

The good news is that by making changes in other areas, you can improve how you feel physically. You will find some helpful advice about how to tackle many of your physical sensations or feelings in the *Overcoming sleep problems* workbook.

Area 5: Your altered behaviour or activity levels

You have already worked hard in thinking about the first four of the five areas in your Five Areas assessment – well done! Here you look at the last area – altered behaviour (things that you can do).

Some things that you do can worsen your feeling of depression. On the other hand, many ways in which you respond can be very helpful and boost how you are. The ways in which your altered behaviours may worsen your low mood or depression are:

- Reducing your activity levels by not doing as much as before.

- Avoiding or escaping from doing things that seem scary or too difficult.

- Starting to respond in ways that backfire and make you feel worse. For example by pushing others away, losing your temper at others for no good reason or having too much alcohol to block how you feel.

All these changes can worsen how you feel.

Key point

Making changes in your behaviour and activity levels are some of the most helpful things you can do to boost how you feel.

First type of altered behaviour: Reduced activity

When you feel down, it's hard to keep doing things because you have:

- Low energy and feel tired ('I'm too tired').
- Little sense of enjoyment or achievement when you do things.
- Negative thoughts about things ('I just can't be bothered').

All these lead to reduced activity – where you do less of, or stop, doing things **which are important** to you. Often the first things that are squeezed out are things that have previously given you a sense of fun or achievement (for example, meeting up with friends, and talking and playing with your baby). You can also lose your sense of closeness to others.

It begins to feel as though everything is too much effort. And so you feel worse and worse.

Your reduced activities

Q Has the depression caused you to:

- Cut down or stop everyday life activities you used to enjoy?

  Yes ☐   No ☐   Sometimes ☐

- Reduce or remove things from life that previously gave you a sense of pleasure/achievement?

  Yes ☐   No ☐   Sometimes ☐

- Reduce or stop doing things that gave you a sense of closeness to others?

  Yes ☐   No ☐   Sometimes ☐

- Overall, has this worsened how you feel?

  Yes ☐   No ☐   Sometimes ☐

Write down any examples here:

The good news is that once you have noticed whether this is true for you, then you can start working on your reduced activity in a planned, step-by-step way. You will find out how to do this in the workbook *Doing things that boost how you feel.*

Second type of altered behaviour: Avoiding or escaping from things

We often start to avoid or escape from people, places and situations that worry us. Such behaviour may make you feel less anxious in the short term. But in the longer term, avoiding things makes it harder and harder to confidently face your fears in the future. And you don't see that your worst fears don't actually occur. In fact, avoidance teaches us the unhelpful rule that we only coped with a situation by avoiding it.

Key point

Avoidance and escaping can make you feel worse and also undermine your confidence.

Some things you may be avoiding

- Breastfeeding when others may see.

- Asking for help when you could do with some.

- Going out.

- Talking about how low you're feeling.

Avoiding or escaping from people, places and situations that worry you

Q Have your depression or anxious feelings caused you to avoid people, places or situations?

Yes ☐   No ☐   Sometimes ☐

If you answered 'Yes' or 'Sometimes':

- Has this reduced your confidence in things?

Yes ☐   No ☐   Sometimes ☐

- Has your life become increasingly restricted?

  Yes ☐   No ☐   Sometimes ☐

- Are you avoiding conversations you need to have?

  Yes ☐   No ☐   Sometimes ☐

- Overall, has this worsened how you feel?

  Yes ☐   No ☐   Sometimes ☐

Write down any examples here:

Key point

The good news is that once you have noticed if this is true for you, you can start working on tackling avoidance and escaping. You need to do this in a planned, step-by-step way. The workbook *Anxiety and avoidance* tells you how to do this.

Third type of altered behaviour: Dropping helpful things you do

Helpful behaviours include doing things such as:

- Talking to friends or family for support, and yet being firm about when you need to sort things out yourself without other people taking over.

- Recognising the times when you have been too hard on yourself.

- Reading or using self-help materials or attending a self-help group to find out more about the causes and treatment of postnatal depression.

- Going to see a doctor or healthcare practitioner to discuss whether you need extra help.

- Finding activities or meeting people – things that you can do with your baby. Preferably think of things that give you pleasure, or a feeling of achievement or closeness to other people.

- If you have a personal spiritual faith, your beliefs may provide helpful support.

My helpful behaviours

Q Has the depression caused you to stop doing activities that help you?

Yes ☐   No ☐   Sometimes ☐

If you answered 'Yes' or 'Sometimes':

● Is this worsening how you feel?

Yes ☐   No ☐   Sometimes ☐

Write down any examples here:

You can find out more about the different ways of building helpful responses in the workbooks *Helpful things you do* and *Doing things that boost how you feel*.

Fourth type of altered behaviour: Unhelpful things you do

Sometimes people may do things that make them feel better at first but in the longer term, these things backfire and make you feel worse. Do you do any of the following unhelpful behaviours?

● Withdrawing into yourself and cutting yourself off from your friends or family.

● Neglecting yourself (for example, by not eating as much or not washing).

● Finding yourself tempted to do things that you know are unwise or wrong. This might include deliberately taking risks, picking fights or betraying a partner.

● Acting out of frustration or anger to harm or hurt others – that is, acting in ways to test out the love or support of others. For example, being rude and critical, or pushing them away to see how much they really want to support you.

● Using alcohol or street drugs to block how you feel.

- Harming yourself as a way of blocking how you feel (for example, self-cutting).
- Shouting or screaming at your baby out of frustration.

My unhelpful behaviours

Q Has the depression caused you to react in ways to try to make you feel better immediately?

Yes ☐   No ☐   Sometimes ☐

If you answered 'Yes' or 'Sometimes':

- Are you doing any actions that make you or others feel worse now or later?

Yes ☐   No ☐   Sometimes ☐

Write down any examples here:

Key point

An important thing to watch out for is whether you have got into a habit of reacting to difficult situations in these ways. By watching out for any unhelpful behaviours that you may have a tendency to fall into, and by choosing to respond differently, you can make large changes in how you are feeling.

You will find out more about reducing unhelpful behaviours in the workbook *Unhelpful things you do*.

Summary for Area 5: Your altered behaviour or activity levels

Now think about all the altered behaviours you have identified and rate the extent of your problems in this area.

No problems at all   The worst they could possibly be

0	1	2	3	4	5	6	7	8	9	10

The Five Areas and your baby

You have now spent quite a lot of time learning about how low mood can affect you in each of the Five Areas. Now use this same approach to think through how depression can also affect your relationship with your baby and those around you.

Area 1: People and events around you

You may feel alone, and that no-one is supporting you. Understandably, when you have a baby, you may focus more on them. Your friends and even your partner may be squeezed out of the picture. Because you aren't following your usual routines, you may not have the same money or social life you had before.

Area 2: Your thinking

You may be very critical of yourself and feel as if you aren't being a good mother. You may become very sensitive to other people's comments and think that they are judging you badly. You may have lots of worrying thoughts about your own abilities as a mother, or about your child's safety and health.

Area 3: Your feelings/emotions

You may not feel about the baby in the way you thought you would. For example many women who have postnatal depression feel nothing for their baby, or may even feel resentful towards them or others such as a partner or close relatives. You may feel guilty that you aren't meeting your own high standards.

Area 4: Your altered physical symptoms

Depression can make you feel tired and tense, and you can even feel pain or sleep poorly. This can push some mothers to a state of desperation and a feeling that they can't cope.

Area 5: Any altered behaviour or activity levels

You may have stopped or reduced doings things that previously would have given you a boost. Sometimes new mothers try to push others away and isolate themselves. Or they do things to unhelpfully block how they are feeling, such as smoking or drinking. Or you may obsessively clean the house or feel you must play with or look after your baby all the time. Because of this, many mothers withdraw emotionally from their baby and others. This makes the feelings of failure worse, and also can affect how much time you are spending playing and talking to your baby.

Another workbook – *Building relationships with your baby, family and friends* deals with how you can bring about changes here and also how to build or rebuild relationships.

What next?

Remember that the purpose of the Five Areas Approach is to help you work out how your low mood is affecting you. By helping you recognise how you are feeling now, this approach can help you plan the areas you need to focus on to bring about change.

The good news is that all the areas are linked so that making changes in any one area can lead to change in the others. So if you try to alter any one of these areas, it will help lift your low mood and help you tackle feeling low or stressed.

Where do you start?

The workbooks in this course can help you begin to tackle all of the five problem areas of depression.

Key point

One key to success is to try not to tackle everything at once. You are more likely to improve if you take slow, steady steps than if you are too enthusiastic at the start and then run out of steam. So try to take things one step at a time by choosing which areas you are going to focus on to start with.

Set yourself:

- Short-term targets: these are changes you can make today, tomorrow and next week.
- Medium-term targets: these are changes to be put in place over the next few weeks.
- Long-term targets: this is where you want to be in six months or a year.

Which workbook should you try first?

Your Five Areas assessment will help you choose which workbooks to read first. Pick just one area and one workbook of the course first. This means that you are actively choosing not to focus on the other areas to start with.

Workbook	Plan to read	Tick when completed
Starting out … and how to keep going if you feel stuck	☐	☐
Understanding why you feel as you do	☐	☐
Making changes to do with people and events		
Practical problem solving	☐	☐
Being assertive	☐	☐
Building relationships with your baby, family and friends	☐	☐
Information for families and friends – how can you offer the best support?	☐	☐
Making changes to behaviours and activity levels		
Doing things that boost how you feel	☐	☐
Using exercise to boost how you feel	☐	☐
Helpful things you do	☐	☐
Unhelpful things you do	☐	☐
Anxiety and avoidance	☐	☐
Making changes to negative and upsetting thinking		
Noticing and changing extreme and unhelpful thinking	☐	☐
Making changes to things that affect your bodily well-being		
Overcoming sleep problems	☐	☐
Alcohol, drugs and your baby	☐	☐
Understanding and using antidepressant medication	☐	☐
Making changes for the future		
Planning for the future	☐	☐

If you want help in deciding where to start, we recommend you read the following workbooks first:

- *Doing things that boost how you feel.*

- *Overcoming sleep problems.*

- If you are taking, or thinking of taking, an anti-depressant try reading *Understanding and using anti-depressant medication* as soon as you can.

If you have a close family member or friend you'd like to help you in using the course, ask them to read the *Information for families and friends* workbook. You also may find it helpful.

Key point

Repeat your **Five Areas assessment** after using each workbook to help you decide where to go next.

How do I know if I need extra help?

Ideally anyone using these workbooks will have someone to support them but there are times when this won't be enough. If you struggle to do the tasks in the workbooks, don't worry. Just do what you can. But if things still do not seem to be improving, you may need to get extra help. If you have somebody supporting you, discuss what you have been doing with them. Otherwise make an appointment to see your doctor or a mental health worker.

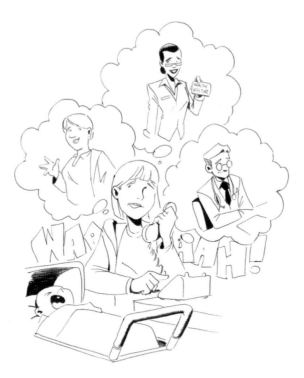

You *really need* to get extra help for:

- **Severe depression**, for example continuing low mood, tearfulness, not eating or drinking much at all or a big loss of weight despite attempts to improve things.

- Strong urges to **self-harm** or feeling really **hopeless or suicidal** about the future.

- Strong urges to harm your baby or anyone else.

- Other **dangerous behaviours**, for example risk-taking, threats of harm to others.

- Not being able to cope so much that you are concerned about the health and well-being of your child or children.

- **Severe withdrawal from life activities**.

Some people have fears that if they admit they are not coping, or are struggling with their baby, that they may lose care of their baby. In fact, mental and social services try their best to help parents look after their children at home. Sharing worries you have about your baby will allow you to get this help.

There can be other situations where extra help might be needed. If either you are (or the person supporting you is) still worried that something else needs to be done, then it is important to ask for help at least in *deciding* whether more help is needed.

Key point

It is better to ask for help or advice than do nothing.

Getting extra help

You can ask:

- **Someone you can trust** – or you may find it easier to talk to someone *outside* your closest friends and family. Don't feel guilty if this is the case, it's actually *normal* to feel like this.

- **Your GP**. He or she can give you medical advice and (if they feel it is necessary) refer you to a specialist mental health worker or team for a fuller assessment.

- **Social services**. They can be a great source of support. Look at your local *Yellow Pages* for the local office hours number and a 24-hour emergency number for initial referrals and queries.

Other organisations/sources you can approach for help are:

- **NSPCC**. You can call the NSPCC adult helpline (0808 800 5000) if you are worried about a child.

- Local counselling services, including **Relate** (**www.relate.org.uk**) – you can call them on 0300 100 1234 for relationship counselling (you need to pay for this).

- **Royal College of Psychiatrists**. You can get fact sheets about postnatal depression by calling 020 7235 2351 or visiting the college's website (**www.rcpsych.ac.uk/mentalhealthinformation/mentalhealthproblems/ postnatalmentalhealth/postnataldepression.aspx**).

Other books that may be of help

- *Overcoming Anxiety: A Five Areas Approach* by Dr C Williams.

- *Overcoming Depression and Low Mood: A Five Areas Approach* by Dr C Williams.

- *I'm Not Supposed to Feel Like This: A Christian Self-help Approach to Depression and Anxiety* by Chris Williams, Paul Richards and Ingrid Whitton.

- *Mind over Mood* by Christine Padesky and Dennis Greenberger.

Short, key skills booklets available from **www.fiveareas.com**:

- Why do I feel so bad?

- How to fix almost everything.

- Why does everything always go wrong?

- I can't be bothered doing anything.

- The things you do that mess you up.

- Are you strong enough to keep your temper (anger).

- I'm not good enough (low confidence).

- 10 things you can do to make you feel happier straight away.

- I feel so bad I can't go on.

- Write all over your bathroom mirror: And 14 other ways to get the most out of your little book (using self-help approaches).

… and others.

 www.livinglifetothefull.com

- This is a free online training course.

- You can download linked handouts as well as teaching exercises to reinforce and build on the changes you have made with the help of these course workbooks.

- The website also has links to an online DVD provided with support from the Scottish Government Health Department that can help you learn key life skills confidentially and for free.

Summary

In this workbook you have:

- Understood what is low mood and depression, and completed a timeline of how your problems have developed.

- Learnt how to complete your own Five Areas assessment to check how you are feeling.

- Learnt how to choose which other course workbooks you should use.

- Learnt when you should get extra help and where to go for it.

Q What have I learnt from this workbook?

Q What do I want to try *next*?

 Task

Write down **three things** that went well every day for a week:

Stop, think and reflect on these points every evening. Why did these things go well? Use these things to find out what were the helpful things you have done that you can build on in your life.

A request for feedback

An important part of the development of this course is that the content is updated on a regular basis, based on feedback from users and practitioners. Please send any feedback that you may have about this workbook to the address given below. You can also email your feedback. However, we can't answer specific questions or provide advice on treatment.

Address: Five Areas, PO Box 9, Glasgow G63 0WL, UK

 Our website: **www.livinglifetothefull.com**
email: **feedback@fiveareas.com**

Acknowledgements

We wish to thank all those who have commented and contributed suggestions used in this workbook, especially Nicky Dummett and Keith Chan.

My notes

PART 2

Making changes

Overcoming Postnatal Depression
A Five Areas Approach

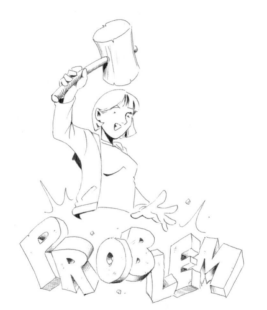

Practical problem solving

www.livinglifetothefull.com
www.fiveareas.com

Dr Chris Williams, Dr Roch Cantwell and
Karen Robertson

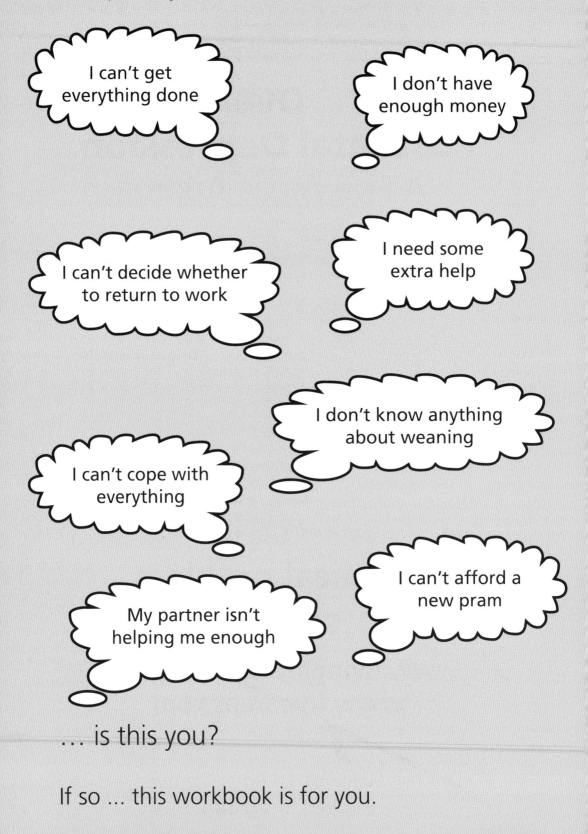

... is this you?

If so ... this workbook is for you.

In this workbook you will:

- Learn how practical problems can affect life.

- Learn to recognise these problems in your own life.

- See an example of problem solving in practice and apply it to a problem of your own.

- Learn how to make slow, steady changes to your life.

How problems affect us

Everyone faces some problems and difficulties in life. It's often easier to cope when there's just one problem. But when you face a particularly hard problem or a whole lot of smaller things all at the same time, you can struggle to cope and feel overwhelmed. This is especially so when you've had a baby.

With a first baby, many parents describe everything as feeling very new and sometimes also scary. Lots of skills such as changing nappies, bathing and breastfeeding or bottle feeding need to be learned. Things don't necessarily seem any smoother when you have a second (or more) baby. You may be much more confident about the practical things, having been through this before, but there are fresh challenges. For example, how will the new baby with no regular routine fit in with the existing routines of older children.

So whether this is your first or another baby, their arrival will dominate your life for a while. There's so much to do, so much to decide. It's understandable then that other life issues take second place. But you know other problems need to be dealt with as well. This workbook will help you achieve this.

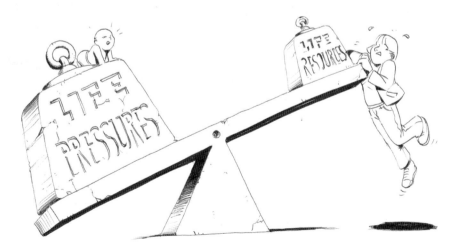

Before you start

Sometimes problems occur because of things we can't control. But sometimes they're the result of things that could have been done differently. For example, problems in relationships may build up because one person ignored a misunderstanding and kept expecting the other person to do something but without making it clear what was needed. Perhaps they didn't respond in ways that would have prevented things worsening at an earlier stage.

Therefore, before you start working on the plan you need to think about these three things:

1. **Your behaviour**: Do you find that the same kinds of problem occur again and again? If so, is there anything that you keep doing (or not doing) that leads to the problem? If you answered 'Yes', you may find the workbook on *Unhelpful things you do* useful.

2. **Your thinking**: Before starting to tackle your practical problems it's important that you choose the right target. So the very first thing to do is to understand whether the problem really is such an issue. Is it possible that things are being blown up out of all proportion because of how you feel at the moment? If you think this may be so, then try reading the *Noticing and changing extreme and unhelpful thinking* workbook to help you get things back into perspective.

3. **Other people and other ways of support**: Some problems are hard to change by yourself. So check out who is there around you whom you could ask for support if you feel you can't do this on your own. Or you may have access to supportive health workers whom you are happy to work with. Even if at the moment you have few or none of these supports, there may be other resources around you that you may have used in the past and helped you feel better. See the list of useful contacts in the *Understanding why you feel as you do* workbook. Also, your GP can help point you to several local supports and aids, so please do discuss problems where you feel stuck and overwhelmed.

Task

Make a list of any practical resources and supports that you have:

At times of distress, people sometimes seem aware of only the problems. You may overlook or downplay your strengths. This can make you ignore the supports you have just listed above, even though they are there. But remember: the supports you have listed may be part of your solution.

How to tackle problems

By approaching your practical problems one step at a time, it is possible to begin tackling them.

- Approach each problem separately, and in turn.
- Define the problem clearly.
- Break down seemingly enormous and unmanageable problems into smaller parts that are then easier to solve.

Having a plan

Setting targets in a planned way can help you to focus on how to make the changes needed to get better. To do this you will need to decide:

- **Short-term** targets – these are changes you can make today, tomorrow and the next week.
- **Medium-term** targets – these are changes you could make over the next few weeks.
- **Long-term** targets – this is where you want to be in six months or a year.

The seven steps to problem solving

Step 1: Identify and clearly define the problem

Overleaf is a list of common practical and relationship problems that happen when you have low mood and depression. Are any of these affecting you? Most mothers face many issues every day, so it's likely that you will have noticed problems in at least some of these areas.

Practical issues	Yes	No	Sometimes
I have worries about money or debts	☐	☐	☐
There are problems where I live	☐	☐	☐
I/somebody close to me doesn't have a job	☐	☐	☐
I/somebody close to me doesn't enjoy their job	☐	☐	☐
I don't have time to do everything needed around the house	☐	☐	☐
I don't have time to do everything needed in my other commitments outside the house/family	☐	☐	☐
There's something I need to buy or borrow	☐	☐	☐
There's too much to do in the available time	☐	☐	☐
There's something practical I don't understand that I need to find out about	☐	☐	☐
There's an item that's broken/damaged/leaking that needs fixing	☐	☐	☐
Relationship issues			
There is no-one around who I can really talk to	☐	☐	☐
I have relationship issues (such as arguments) with my partner/spouse	☐	☐	☐
My partner/spouse doesn't really talk to me or offer me enough support	☐	☐	☐
I have relationship issues (such as arguments) with close family members, for example parents/brother/sister	☐	☐	☐
I'm not spending time with my baby like I want to	☐	☐	☐
My children won't do what I tell them	☐	☐	☐
Someone close to me has alcohol or drug problems	☐	☐	☐
Someone close to me has problems with the police or courts	☐	☐	☐
Someone close to me is being threatened by somebody	☐	☐	☐
There's someone else, like a sick relative, I have to care for	☐	☐	☐
I have difficulties with others, for example neighbours/friends/colleagues at work	☐	☐	☐

Write down any other practical or relationship issues you are facing:

Example: Julia's practical problem

Julia's baby son Ben is now growing out of his Moses basket. Also his pushchair, which was a gift, is beginning to break. She therefore needs to get a cot and a pram, but she doesn't have much money. Julia ticks several boxes in the list of problems, but she decides the one she wants to focus on is: There's something I need to buy or borrow – the cot.

Now it's your turn

Look back at your list and choose **one** problem that you will tackle first. This is particularly important if you have ticked many boxes in the list. It isn't possible to overcome all these problems at once, so you need to decide which **one** area to focus on.

My target area: In the space below write down the one problem area you want to work on first.

Key point

Remember that this should be a practical or relationship problem.

Breaking it down into small steps

The important thing is to use a **step-by step** approach where no step seems too large. And the first step needs to be something that gets you moving in the right direction. For many problems, you may need to break down your target into many smaller steps that you can tackle one at a time.

Example: Julia's step-by-step approach

Julia decides to break down the task – getting the cot – into some smaller steps. This is because she doesn't have enough money to just go out and get one. It needs to be one that's low cost but good enough, and also one they can pick up or have dropped off as they don't have a car. She therefore decides that as a first step she will **try to get one locally at low cost**.

Now decide whether you need to **break your target into smaller steps**.

Q Is this a clear, focused problem I can tackle?

Yes ☐   No ☐

Q Do you need to break it down into smaller, more achievable targets?

Yes ☐   No ☐

If you answered 'Yes', then please go straight to Step 2. If you answered 'No', then keep reading about how to choose a realistic first target.

So think about your problem again. What smaller steps could help you move forwards? If you need to, write down your first target here again.

My clear and realistic first step is:

Step 2: Think up as many solutions as possible to achieve your first goal

When you feel overwhelmed by practical problems, often it's hard to see a way out. It can seem hard to even start tackling the problem.

One way around this is to step back from the problem and see if any other solutions are possible. This approach is called **brainstorming**. The more solutions that you can think of, the more likely it is that a good one will emerge.

Key point

You can even include ridiculous ideas at first as you are just trying to get yourself to start thinking more flexibly!

The purpose of brainstorming is to try to come up with **as many ideas as possible**. Then it will be easier for you to identify the solution that should overcome your problem.

The following questions will help you come up with possible ideas:

● What advice would you give a friend who was trying to make the same changes? Sometimes it's easier to think of solutions for others than for ourselves.

- What *ridiculous* solutions can you include as well as more sensible ones?

- What helpful ideas would others (e.g. family, friends or colleagues) suggest?

- What have you tried in the past that was helpful?

Example: Julia's problem – possible solutions to getting a cot at low cost

(Including ridiculous ideas at first)

- Ignore the problem completely – it may go away.
- I could steal one from somewhere.
- I could go to the local shop and see if there are any adverts up.
- I could look in the local paper/free sheet and see if there's anything available.
- I could ask round my friends and relatives and see if they have one/any ideas.
- I could put a 'Wanted' card up in the newsagent.

Now write down as many possible solutions (including ridiculous ideas at first) for your own problem:

Step 3: Look at the pros and cons of each possible solution

Example: Julia writes down the pros and cons of her solutions

Suggestion	Pros (advantages)	Cons (disadvantages)
Ignore the problem completely – it may go away	Easier in the short term and I don't have to think about it. I might be able to manage without a cot	Well Ben could sleep in a Moses basket for a few more weeks – but not when he's 18! We'll need to get a cot some time soon
I could steal one from somewhere	Well it might work, but ...	I don't want to do that – it's wrong. It's one of my whacky brainstorm ideas. Even if I did think like that I wouldn't. I'd get fined and have even less money than I have now
I could go to the local shop and see if there are any adverts up	That's a good idea – people often advertise lots of stuff at a good price. I might even be able to carry it home as the seller should be local	There might not be one for sale there. Knowing my luck there will be someone else trying to buy a cot as well
I could look in the local paper/free sheet and see if there's anything available	That's another good idea – they have loads of pages with stuff for sale	I'd need to spend time looking through the pages and then follow it up
I could ask round my friends and relatives and see if they have one/any ideas	Lots of them have had children. One of them may have a cot they want to get rid of	I'd have to spend time getting in touch with them all
I could put a 'Wanted' card up in the newsagent	Well, I've seen other people do this. It must work sometimes	I'd feel a bit nervous asking the newsagent if I could put it up. Do you have to pay for that sort of thing?

Write your own list of ideas below, and the pros and cons of each suggestion.

My suggestions from Step 2	Pros (advantages)	Cons (disadvantages)

Step 4: Now choose one of the solutions

In making your decision, bear in mind that the best way of tackling a problem is to plan **steady, slow changes**.

Key point

The solution you are looking for is something that gets you moving in the right direction. This should be small enough to be possible, but big enough to move you forwards.

Example: Julia's final choice

- Julia tries to choose an option that will make a sensible first step in achieving her goal. She knows her chosen solution should be realistic and then it will be likely to succeed. She makes her decision after looking at all the pros and cons she's listed in Step 3.
- Julia decides on balance to first **ask her friends and relatives**. Many of the other suggestions might also work, but this suggestion seems a reasonable first step.

Look at your own responses in Step 3 and then choose a solution. Write down your preferred option here:

Now see if you can answer 'Yes' to the first three **Questions for effective change** below.

Q Will it be *useful* for changing how you are?

Yes ☐   No ☐

 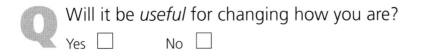

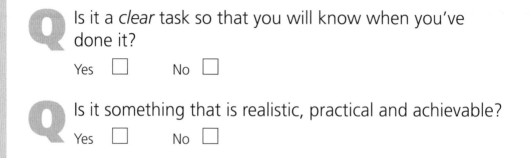

Is it a *clear* task so that you will know when you've done it?

Yes ☐   No ☐

Is it something that is realistic, practical and achievable?

Yes ☐   No ☐

If you answered 'Yes' to all three questions your chosen step should help start you off. If you answered 'No', then think again and choose another option from your list.

Step 5: Plan the steps needed to carry out your chosen solution

You need to have a clear plan that lays out exactly **what** you are going to do and **when** you are going to do it. *Write down* the steps needed to carry out your plan. This will help you to think what to do and also to predict possible problems that might arise. Remember that an important part of the planning process is to predict what would block the plan. That way you can think about how you will respond if there were problems keeping your plan on track.

Example: Julia's plan

Who do I know? I know my sister's using her cot so that won't do. That cot came from my parents – they never throw anything away – but they only had one. I think I need to ask my friends.

So I'll ask Emma, she knows everyone, and also Mark – he's a bit of a wheeler-dealer. He might be able to find something. And I'll also ask my friend Sarah. She works next door to a charity shop and she could have a look out for me. I'll phone them just now while Ben is sleeping. Now, let's think. Is that a plan that makes clear what I'm going to do and when I'm going to do it? – Yes it is. I don't think this will be blocked or prevented by anything – unless Ben wakes up! If so I'll phone later. If this doesn't work within a few days I can always go back to my brainstorm at Step 2 and go to the local shop to put up the advert.

Now, write down your plan here:

 What will you do if something happens that may block your plan?

Write down what you could do to unblock your plan:

Now check your plan against the rest of the **Questions for effective change**.

Q Is your plan one that:

- Makes clear what you are going to do and when you are going to do it?

  Yes ☐   No ☐

- Won't be easily blocked or prevented by practical problems?

  Yes ☐   No ☐

- Will help you to learn useful things even if it doesn't work out perfectly?

  Yes ☐   No ☐

Step 6: Carry out your plan

Now carry out your plan during the next week.

Good luck!

Step 7: Review the outcome

Example 1: If Julia's plan works

Julia carries out her plan. She phones the people she knows and they all promise to help. She thinks she won't hear anything back for a few days – but then just two hours later Emma phones back. Julia knows that Emma knows everybody and everybody knows Emma. Emma says she has been chatting to a friend whose youngest child has just moved into a bed. They now have no need or space for the cot – in fact they were beginning to worry about how to get rid of it because they don't have a car. They have told Emma that if Julia can pick it up then she can have it for free. Emma and Julia both feel very pleased. The plan worked.

Example 2: If Julia's plan doesn't work

Julia carries out her plan. She phones the people she knows and they all promise to help. But after four days no-one has phoned back. Julia is disappointed, but she already knows what she will do now (her back-up plan). She will put an advertisement in a local shop. She then plans what to do (see Step 5 on page 66). She asks her friend Emma to come to the shop with her (for moral support). They find out that putting the advertisement up is free. The adverts are put on the wall next to the till where people queue. Two days later Julia gets a call from someone who is willing to sell them a cot at a good price.

Now write down your review here:

Was your plan successful?

Yes ☐   No ☐

Did it help improve things?

Yes ☐   No ☐

Did any problems arise?

Yes ☐   No ☐

What have you learned from doing this?

Write down any helpful lessons or information you have learned from what happened. If things didn't go quite as you hoped, try to learn from this.

 ## How could you make things different during your next attempt to tackle the problem?

 ## Were you too ambitious or unrealistic in choosing the target you did?

If you noticed problems with your plan

Choosing realistic targets for change is important. Think back to where you started – were you too ambitious or unrealistic in choosing the target you did? Sometimes your attempt to solve a problem may be blocked by something unexpected. Perhaps something didn't happen as you planned, or someone reacted in an unexpected way? Try to learn from what happened.

 How could you change how you approach the problem to help you make a realistic action plan?

Planning the next steps

After completing the first step you need to plan another change to build on this. You will need to slowly build on what you have done in a step-by-step way.

Did your plan help you completely tackle the problem you were working on? You may need to plan out other solutions to tackle different aspects of your problem. The important thing is to build one step upon another.

So you now have the choice to:

- Focus on the same problem area and plan to keep working on it one step at a time.

- Choose a new problem area to work on.

Steps should always be realistic, practical and achievable. Without a step-by-step approach you may find that although you take some steps forward, these can be all in different directions. So you could lose your focus and motivation. Use what you have just learned to build on what you did.

Example: Julia's next steps

I've now found a cot, but it's in a flat three miles away on the estate. We don't have a car – how can we go and get it?

Julia then creates a new seven-step plan. She asks her friends from next door, who have a car, if they can help. They drive over together and pick up the cot. She and her partner Dave make it up in Ben's bedroom and are delighted. That night Ben sleeps in his own room for the first time.

Julia has now sorted out her problem and has the new cot she wanted. Now it's your turn. When making your next plan:

Do:

- Plan to work on **only** one or two key problems over the next week.

- Plan to alter things slowly in a step-by-step way.

- Use the **Questions for effective change** to check that the next step is always well planned.

- Write down your plan in detail so that you know exactly what you are going to do this week.

Don't:

- Try to start to alter too many things all at once.

- Choose something that is too hard a target to start with.

- Be negative and think 'It's a waste of time'. Try to find out if this negative thinking is actually true.

Write your own short, medium and long-term plans here:

- **Short term** – what might you do over the next week or so? This is your next step you need to plan.

- **Medium term** – what might you aim towards doing over the next few weeks – the next few steps?

- **Longer term** – where do you want to be in a few months or so?

Remember to plan slow, steady changes. By breaking down problems and tackling them one step at a time any problem can be addressed.

When you need more help

Remember, you are not alone. If you need more help consider asking:

- People around you, who you know and trust

- Your GP, health visitor or social worker.

A longer list of supports is provided at the end of the *Understanding why you feel as you do* and the *Planning for the future* workbooks.

Summary

In this workbook you have:

- Learnt how practical problems affect your life.

- Learnt how to identify problems in your own life that you can change.

- Seen an example of problem solving in practice and have applied this to one of your own problems.

- Learnt how to make slow, steady changes to your life.

 What have I learnt from this workbook?

 What do I want to try *next*?

Putting what you have learnt into practice

Continue to put into practice what you learn over the next few weeks. Don't try to solve every problem all at once. Plan out what to do at a pace that's right for you. Build changes one step at a time.

Use the blank summary sheet at the end of the workbook to help you plan your changes. If you are stuck or unsure what to do discuss this with someone else.

Key point

Don't put off asking for help if you are stuck.

 You can print out a small flashcard of the seven steps to problem solving for free at **www.fiveareas.com**

My notes

The seven steps to practical problem solving worksheet

By working through the seven steps in this workbook you will learn an approach that will help you to solve your problems.

Step 1: Identify and clearly define the problem

Select the problem area you will tackle.

Do you need to break it down into a smaller target – that is more practical, realistic and achievable in the next week or so? If yes, write down your new target here:

Step 2: Think up as many solutions as possible to achieve your first goal

Brainstorm

What advice would you give a friend? Include ridiculous ideas as well. What have others said? What would you say in five years' time?

Step 3: Look at the pros and cons of each possible solution

Write down a list of the pluses and minuses of each option.

My suggestions from Step 2	Pros (advantages)	Cons (disadvantages)

Step 4: Now choose one of the solutions

Use your answers in Step 3 to make this choice.

My solution

Step 5: Plan the steps needed to carry out your chosen solution

(You'll need to use another sheet of paper for this.)

Apply the **Questions for effective change**.

Q Is the planned activity one that:

● Will be useful for understanding or changing how you are?

Yes ☐ No ☐

● Is a specific task so that you will know when you have done it?

Yes ☐ No ☐

● Is realistic, practical and achievable?

Yes ☐ No ☐

● Makes clear *what* you are going to do and *when* you are going to do it?

Yes ☐ No ☐

● Is an activity that won't be easily blocked or prevented by practical problems?

Yes ☐ No ☐

● Will help you to learn useful things even if it doesn't work out perfectly?

Yes ☐ No ☐

Add a plan of what you will do if your solution **doesn't fully work out.**

Step 6: Carry out your plan

Step 7: Review the outcome

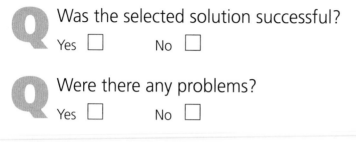

Was the selected solution successful?

Yes ☐   No ☐

Were there any problems?

Yes ☐   No ☐

Q What have you learned from the situation?

Even if the plan wasn't completely successful, there will be things you will have learnt. How can you put what you have learned into practice?

My notes

Overcoming Postnatal Depression
A Five Areas Approach

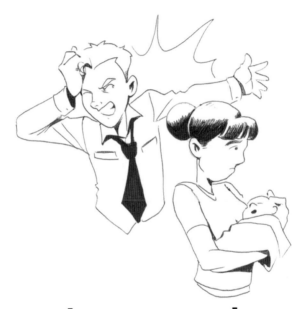

Being assertive

www.livinglifetothefull.com
www.fiveareas.com

Dr Chris Williams, Dr Roch Cantwell and
Karen Robertson

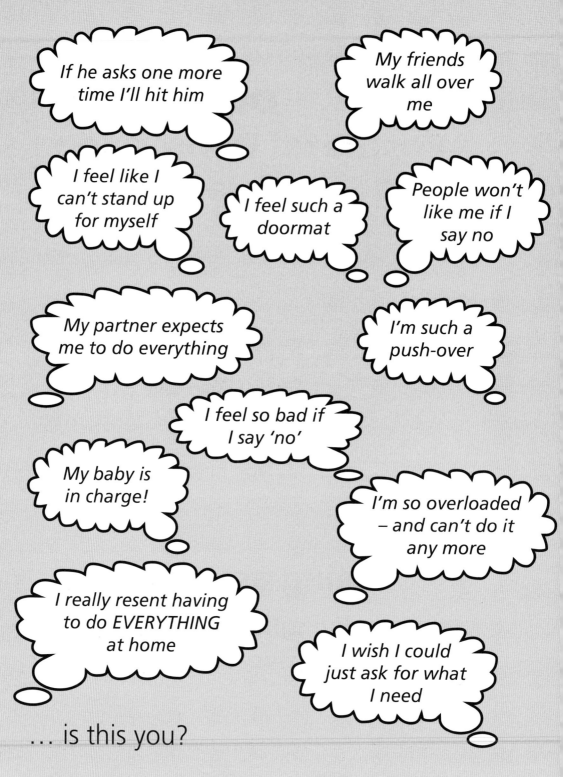

... is this you?

If so ... this workbook is for you.

© Dr Chris Williams (2009)

In this workbook you will:

● Learn about the differences between passive behaviour, aggressive behaviour and assertive behaviour.

● Learn the rules of assertion and how you can put them into practice in everyday situations.

What is assertiveness?

Assertiveness is being able to:

● Stand up for yourself.

● Make sure your opinions and feelings are considered.

● Not let other people always get their way.

Key point

You can be assertive without being forceful or rude.

So assertiveness means stating clearly what you expect and making sure that what you want is considered **as well as** what other people want.

You can **learn and practise** being assertive. By practising being assertive, you'll become more aware of your own needs as an individual.

What do you do in difficult situations?

However confident you are, there are times when one finds it hard to deal with certain situations. For example:

● Dealing with unhelpful shop assistants.

● Planning to have *you* time away from your baby.

● Asking for help with your baby when you need it.

● Asking someone to return something they have borrowed.

● Reacting to people who criticise the way you look after your baby.

- Letting your family or friends know how you feel and what you need.

- Saying no to other people's demands.

Do you deal with these situations by losing your temper, by saying nothing or by **giving in**? If you do, have you noticed that it can leave you feeling unhappy, angry or out of control? And that it may not have actually solved your problem?

How can you become more assertive?

While growing up, people learn to relate to others from their parents, teachers and friends. You may also be influenced by other things such as television and magazines. You may have read about how important it is to be a 'perfect' mother and do a great job all the time. But in trying to do this, you can become so focused on doing things for other people that you may forget to do things for yourself as well.

Sometimes your confidence can get worn away. For example if someone has been bullied or ridiculed when they were growing up, or is criticised a lot by their family. In these situations, you may learn to **react passively or aggressively to people and situations**.

Key point

The good news is that although you may have learned to react passively or aggressively in life, you can become more assertive by learning **assertiveness skills**.

Key elements of passive behaviour

Behaving passively means:

- Always saying 'Yes'.

- Not letting others know about your feelings, needs, rights and opinions.

- Always choosing others' needs over your own.

Usually people behave passively to **avoid conflict** at all times and to **please others**. This kind of behaviour is driven by a fear of not wanting to upset others or have others not like us. But in the longer term, this can make you feel worse.

When someone behaves passively it can cause others to become irritated and have a lack of respect for the person behaving passively. When you behave passively, others can take you for granted and increasingly expect you to drop everything to help them.

Key elements of aggressive behaviour

Aggression is the opposite of assertion.

Behaving aggressively means:

- Not having respect for other people.
- Demanding things in an angry or threatening way. For example, when a new mother, who has been feeling stressed and upset looking after her baby the whole day, launches into a tirade as soon as her partner comes home from work feeling tired and just wanting to relax.
- Thinking your own needs are more important than those of others. An aggressive person ignores other people's needs and thinks they have little or nothing to contribute.

The aim of aggression is to win, even at the expense of others.

Task

Try to think of a time when someone else has been aggressive towards you and ignored your opinions. How did it make you feel about them and yourself?

Overall, in the longer term, being aggressive causes problems for the person being aggressive and for the people around them.

Key point

Behaving aggressively or being passive can be changed by learning the skill of 'assertive behaviour'.

Key elements of assertive behaviour

Assertiveness means:

- Letting others know about your feelings, needs, rights and opinions while maintaining respect for other people.
- Expressing your feelings in a direct, honest and appropriate way.
- Realising it's possible to stand up for your rights in such a way that you don't disregard another person's rights at the same time.

Assertion is **not about winning** but about being able to walk away feeling that you put across what you wanted to say.

 Task

Try to think about a time when someone else has been assertive with you and respected your opinion. How did you feel about them and yourself?

About me – I felt:

About them – I felt:

Benefits of being assertive

Assertiveness is an **attitude** towards yourself and others that is helpful and honest. When you are being assertive, you ask for what you want:

- Directly and openly.

- Appropriately, respecting everyone's opinions and rights, and expecting others to do the same.

- Confidently, without undue anxiety.

By being assertive, you try not to:

- Disregard other people's rights.

- Expect other people to magically know what you want.

- Freeze with anxiety and avoid problems.

Being assertive improves your self-confidence and others' respect for you.

The rules of assertion

The following 12 rules can help you live your life more assertively.

I have the right to:

1. Respect myself – who I am and what I do.

2. Recognise my own needs as an individual, that is, separate from what's expected of me in particular roles, such as 'mother', 'sister, 'partner', 'daughter', 'wife'.

3. Make clear 'I' statements about how I feel and what I think, for example 'I feel very uncomfortable with your decision'.

4. Allow myself to make mistakes, recognising that it's normal to make mistakes.

5. Change my mind, if I choose.

6. Ask for 'thinking about it time'. For example, when people ask you to do something, you have the right to say 'I would like to think it over and I will let you know by the end of the week'.

7. Allow myself to enjoy my successes, that is, being pleased with what I've done and sharing it with others.

8. Ask for what I want, rather than hoping someone will notice what I want.

9. Recognise that I am not responsible for the behaviour of other adults or for pleasing other adults all the time.

10. Respect other people and their right to be assertive and expect the same in return.

11. Say I don't understand.

12. Deal with others without depending on them for approval.

 At the moment, how much do you believe in each of these 12 rules, and do you put them into practice?

I have the right to:	Do I believe this rule is true?		Have I applied this in the last week?	
1. Respect myself	Yes ☐	No ☐	Yes ☐	No ☐
2. Recognise my own needs as an individual independent of others	Yes ☐	No ☐	Yes ☐	No ☐
3. Make clear 'I' statements about how I feel and what I think, for example 'I feel very uncomfortable with your decision'	Yes ☐	No ☐	Yes ☐	No ☐
4. Allow myself to make mistakes	Yes ☐	No ☐	Yes ☐	No ☐
5. Change my mind	Yes ☐	No ☐	Yes ☐	No ☐
6. Ask for 'thinking about it time'	Yes ☐	No ☐	Yes ☐	No ☐
7. Allow myself to enjoy my successes	Yes ☐	No ☐	Yes ☐	No ☐
8. Ask for what I want, rather than hoping someone will notice what I want	Yes ☐	No ☐	Yes ☐	No ☐
9. Recognise that I am not responsible for the behaviour of others or for pleasing others all the time	Yes ☐	No ☐	Yes ☐	No ☐
10. Respect other people and their right to be assertive and expect the same in return	Yes ☐	No ☐	Yes ☐	No ☐
11. Say I don't understand	Yes ☐	No ☐	Yes ☐	No ☐
12. Deal with others without being dependent on them for approval	Yes ☐	No ☐	Yes ☐	No ☐

You can put these rights into practice to develop assertiveness skills by using many assertiveness techniques. Some of these are described below.

Before learning assertiveness techniques, it's important to know how to start a conversation.

Starting and maintaining conversations

Sometimes you can feel isolated if there is no-one around to talk to. You may feel lonely but you lack contact with anyone. There are many practical things you can do to begin to meet people. For example:

- Making friends through people you know already.
- Joining a toddler group, mums and tots, a playgroup or a leisure centre.
- Doing a course or joining a club, for example at your local community hall.
- Visiting other local places, for example community organisations or the local place of worship. Some local shops such as post offices, pharmacies and hairdressers also provide a place to talk.
- Getting in touch with people you know but haven't seen for a while. Use email, write a letter or telephone to get in touch. Arrange to meet if you can.

Here are some good conversation starters:

- How are you?
- Nice day, isn't it?
- Hi, I'm new here and a little bit nervous.
- How old is your baby? He looks so alert.

Key point

Remember – it doesn't matter if you talk about superficial things to begin with, such as the weather, the local news or about the weekend.

You don't have to do this if you don't like it. Instead you can think of some **conversation starters in advance**. Good opening questions often begin with the words:

- **What** – what was mums and tots like last week? What did you do yesterday?
- **How** – how did you find the meal? How are you? How are you getting on with her early waking?

- **When** – when will we be covering this on the course? When did you start her on solids?

- **Who** – who came yesterday? Who's that over there?

- **Why** – why does that happen (or not happen)? Why do we do things this way? Why do they need yet another fundraiser at play group?

Follow these with **back-up questions**. For example:

- Who came yesterday – did they enjoy it?

- What did they say?

- Did it go well?

- Do you think they'll come back?

Assertiveness techniques you could use

Once you get into conversation, the following assertive techniques will help you to build assertive communication into what you say.

'Broken record'

This works in virtually any situation. First, practise what you want to say by repeating over and over again what you want or need. During the conversation, keep returning to your prepared lines, stating clearly what it is you need or want. Do not be put off by clever arguments or by what the other person says. Once you have prepared the lines you want to say, you can relax. Nothing can defeat this tactic!

> ### Example of broken record: Being firm about what you want
>
> Sally: Can you please take Jack upstairs and get him bathed and ready for bed? I have to get the meal ready before you go out to meet your friends in the pub.
>
> John: I can't do that just now – I'm watching the football match.
>
> Sally: I have to get the meal ready before you go out. You can record the match and watch it some other time.
>
> John: But I want to watch the match now.
>
> Sally: I have to get the meal ready before you go out. You can watch the match some other time.
>
> John: Okay then – I'll watch it later when I get back in. But don't tell me the score.

Remember

- Work out beforehand what you want to say.
- Repeat your reply over and over again and stick to what you have decided to say.

Saying 'no'

Many people find that 'no' seems to be one of the hardest words to say. Try to remember when you may have found yourself in situations that you didn't want to be in just because you had avoided saying this one simple word.

Why does this happen? It may be that the images you associate with saying 'no' may prevent you using the word when you need it. People often worry that they may be seen as being mean and selfish, or they may worry about being rejected by others.

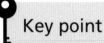

Key point

Saying 'no' can be both important and helpful.

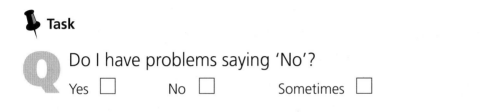 **Task**

Do I have problems saying 'No'?

Yes ☐   No ☐   Sometimes ☐

If you ticked 'Yes' or 'Sometimes', try to practise saying 'No' by using the following techniques:

- Be straightforward and honest so that you can make your point effectively. This isn't the same as being rude.

- Tell the person if you are finding it hard.

- Don't apologise and give all sorts of reasons for saying 'No'. It is okay to say 'No' if you don't want to do things.

- Remember that it is better in the long run to be truthful than breed resentment and bitterness within yourself.

Body language and assertiveness

How people communicate involves more than just words. Your voice tone, how quickly and loudly you speak, eye contact and body posture – all affect how you come over. When you're being assertive be aware of the non-verbal communications you make as well as the words you say.

Eye contact

- Meet the other person's eyes from time to time.

- Make eye contact – but don't end up staring at the person.

- Try not to look down for long – this may look odd or rude to others.

If you find this hard to do, practise looking just past the person. For example, look at a thing such as a picture on the wall behind them.

Your voice

- Try to vary your tone so you come over well.

- Don't be afraid of silence. Remember that small pauses in a conversation can seem long and uncomfortable when you feel anxious. So when you ask a question you may be tempted to fill any uncomfortable gaps yourself. Knowing this can be useful so that you are prepared to allow a little silence. Likewise, you don't need to reply instantly to any question. Remember that you're allowed some time to think.

- Think about how quickly or loudly you talk. If you're anxious or angry you may either speed up and gabble words, or slow down so you come over as hesitant. Either extreme will affect how you come over. Aim for a relaxed yet serious manner if you can.

Posture

Think about how you hold your body:

- Try looking up and don't hunch over – this can happen when you feel vulnerable or anxious.

- Keep an appropriate distance ('personal space') between you and the other person.

- Don't get too close or this might be seen as aggressive or inappropriate (unless you know the person very well).

Be friendly

Smiling once in a while is okay.

Be relaxed in your body

- Again, think about how you hold your body. If you're tense or anxious you may clench your fists and frown, which may come over as being aggressive.

- Relax your body. Quickly screen how you're holding your arms and shoulders and try to relax tense muscles.

A word of caution

Don't think you have to suddenly get all of this right straight away. You should make these changes slowly – over many weeks or even months.

You shouldn't get confused because you are too concerned about things like whether you are avoiding eye contact enough. All you need to do is be aware of this and try to occasionally make some small changes in what you do. Experiment and see what works for you.

Trying out being more assertive

Think about the following when you plan to respond assertively. Choose:

- **The right person**. Some people can take even assertive feedback badly. If you know that what you say is likely to be misinterpreted, or that the person will over-react, then you need to get some extra help, such as from a close friend or a family member.

- **The right time**. For example, try not to start talking about important things as soon as your partner gets in from work or from an evening out. Choose a more relaxed time – or plan such a time – for example go for a walk together.

- **The right issue**. The issue needs be something that the other person can change. For example, asking your mother to look after your baby at times when she has to go to work is not realistic. Instead, discuss a time that will suit you both.

- **The right words**. Use the approaches described in this workbook ('Broken record' and 'Saying no'). These techniques will help you to say what you need.

 Task

Think about how you can be more assertive in your own life. If you recognise that you lack assertiveness, try to:

- Use one of the two assertiveness techniques during the next week.

- Remind yourself about and put into practice the **rules of assertion**. Copy page 90 or tear it out and carry it around with you. Put it somewhere you will see it (for example, by your television or on a door or mirror or on the fridge) to remind you of these rules.

 Credit card-sized versions of the rules of assertion and the seven steps to problem solving are available for you to print for free or order from the Five Areas website (**www.fiveareas.com**).

Summary

In this workbook you have learnt:

- The differences between passive behaviour, aggressive behaviour and assertive behaviour.

- About the rules of assertion and how you can put them into practice in everyday life.

Q What have I learnt from this workbook?

Q What do I want to try *next*?

Putting into practice what you have learned

Read again what you learned earlier in the workbook about the 'Broken record' and 'Saying no' approaches, and try to put them into practice during the next week.

View this as an action plan that can help you to change how you are and also to learn something new about yourself and other people.

My notes

Overcoming Postnatal Depression

A Five Areas Approach

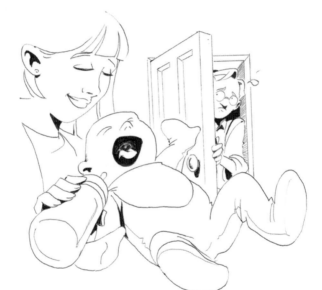

Building relationships with your baby, family and friends

www.livinglifetothefull.com
www.fiveareas.com

Dr Chris Williams, Dr Roch Cantwell and
Karen Robertson

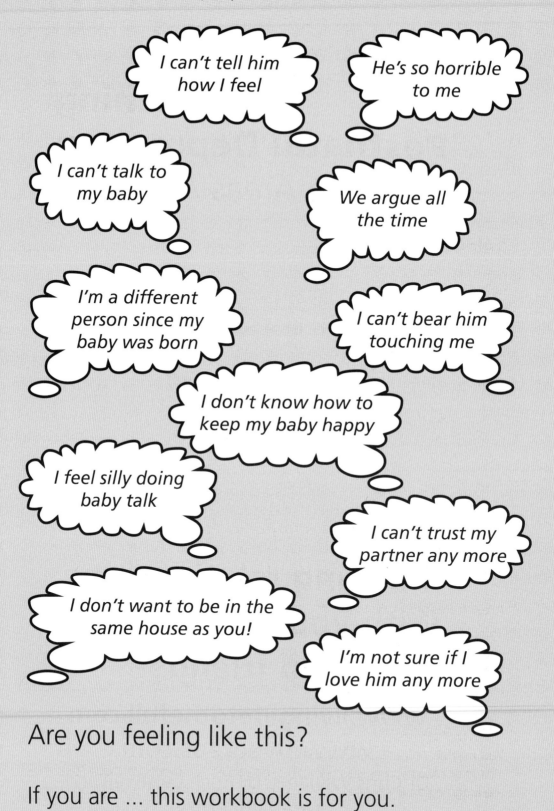

Are you feeling like this?

If you are ... this workbook is for you.

In this workbook you will:

- Review your own style of communicating with others.

- Learn how to play, enjoy and build a loving relationship with your baby.

- Learn how to build (and rebuild) close relationships with the people around you.

- Find out how to develop a new identity as a mother – which includes your old friends.

Relating to your baby

New parents have all sorts of expectations of what things will be like when their baby is born. Having a baby is often a huge adjustment for all involved. If you've just had your first baby, you may feel out of your depth or even scared by all the new information and practical skills you suddenly need to know. Your expectations will also be affected by what you have seen and experienced yourself in your own upbringing, with close friends and relatives who have had children and with information you may pick up from television and magazines.

In the workbook *Understanding why you feel as you do*, you learnt about how postnatal depression can affect the five key areas of your life.

The five areas and your baby

You have now spent quite a lot of time learning about how low mood can affect you in each of the five areas of your life. Now use this same approach to think through how your depression can affect your relationships with your baby and those around you.

Area 1: People and events around you

You may feel alone and that no-one is supporting you. Understandably, when you have a baby, you may focus more on them. Your friends and even your partner may be squeezed out of the picture. Because you aren't following your usual routines, you may not have the same money or social life you had before.

Area 2: Altered thinking

You may be very critical of yourself and feel as if you aren't a good mother. You may become very sensitive to other people's comments and think that they are judging you badly. You may think that other people are better at meeting your baby's needs. You may have lots of worrying thoughts about your own abilities as a mother, or about your child's safety and health.

Area 3: Altered feelings (also called moods or emotions)

You may not feel about the baby in the way you thought you would. For example, many women who have postnatal depression feel nothing for their baby, or may even feel resentful towards them or others such as a partner or close relatives. You may feel guilty that you aren't meeting your own high standards.

Area 4: Altered physical symptoms

Depression can make you feel tired and tense, and you can even feel pain or sleep poorly. This can push some mothers to a state of desperation and a feeling that they cannot cope.

Area 5: Altered behaviour or activity levels

You may have stopped or reduced doing things that previously would have given you a boost. Sometimes new mothers try to push others away and isolate themselves, or do things to unhelpfully block how they are feeling, such as smoking or drinking. Or you may obsessively clean the house or feel you must play or look after your baby all the time and not accept help from others.

Thinking about these five areas will help you understand why your relationship with your baby can be affected. You may feel distanced and a lack of love, and begin to withdraw as a result. It's important to remember that as a parent you have a responsibility to encourage and help your baby to grow and develop. You want your baby to be healthy, to be able to learn and achieve goals, to be able to communicate, to be confident, to eventually be responsible and independent and enjoy their own relationships with other people. By building a loving and nurturing relationship with your baby, you will help these things happen in their life. When you are depressed, this responsibility can feel overwhelming.

However, there are some very simple things that you can do to help your baby grow and develop.

Building a loving relationship with your baby

Communicating

Babies start trying to communicate as soon as they are born. They can't use speech but they will pull faces, cry, scream, smile, yawn, gurgle, stare and make garbled noises. When they cry, they are looking for their carer – usually their mother – to feed, change, wind or cuddle them. You may feel silly talking to your baby when they can't speak back, but they will thrive on you looking at their eyes, smiling and talking to them. You can try 'taking turns' for example. If your baby pulls a face or smiles, copy what they are doing back to them. Then you start communicating with them by pulling a face or smiling – and watch as your baby copies you. You should try to talk to your baby as you go about your day-to-day tasks. Even though your baby won't understand what you are saying, the interaction will help their development.

Sometimes when your baby looks away from you when you are talking to them, you might think they don't like you, or that you are boring them. But this isn't the case! Because your baby's brain is developing at a fast pace, it needs time to process the information it is taking in, and for this reason, it's normal for your baby to break eye contact with you for a few moments.

Play, encouragement and fun

Playing with your baby doesn't have to be hard. You can do very simple things that your baby will enjoy, while also learning at the same time. You don't have to play with your baby all day long, but it's good to play for 20 minutes or so a few times every day. You can do this while you are attending to their everyday care needs. This might be when you are bathing your baby or changing their nappy, or even after they have just woken up from a sleep.

Here are some ideas for how you can play with your baby:

- Play a game of peek-a-boo.
- Sing nursery rhymes, gently clapping their hands.
- Read them a story, even if they are too young to speak.
- Encourage them by praising them as they learn to reach out and clasp or hold something, or learn to clap their hands.

You don't need to have lots of expensive toys for your baby to play with. They will get just as much fun from home-made toys such as banging a plastic spoon on a plastic tub, or using colourful plastic cups to play with water in the bath. Your local library may have a toy library as well as books for all ages. Babies and children can also have their own library card.

Remember you are an important person in your baby's life. They need you to help them grow and develop. Your baby will not judge you or criticise you. As you communicate, play and care for your baby, your relationship with them will build over time. You will feel more confident and at ease with them, and begin to enjoy being with them.

Relating to other adults

We are all different. Some of us have many friends and acquaintances. Others prefer to keep themselves to themselves and have fewer people around who are 'close'. Whatever sort of style of relationship you prefer, your relationships will alter after having a baby, especially if you have postnatal depression.

Our past and present relationships are some of the most powerful factors that affect how we feel. You have already seen in the *Being assertive* workbook how early relationships influence the way in which you relate to others now. Remember that people tend to repeat the pattern or styles of relating that they learn in childhood. For example, during your upbringing, you learned important rules about:

- How you should communicate with others – with assertiveness, passivity or aggression.

- How you expect others to relate to you – whether they are trustworthy or will let you down.

Many of the rules people learn are helpful and positive. For example that you are loved, trusted and accepted. However, sometimes the rules are more negative and unhelpful.

Key point

Most of us learn a mixture of both helpful and unhelpful rules and these can affect how you react and trust others – especially when you are upset.

Now use the checklist below to find out your own styles of relating.

What you may have learnt from past experience	How this affects your relationships now (your relationship style)	Tick here if this applies to you – even if only sometimes
Learning generally positive things about how you see yourself, others and relationships You have a reasonable self-esteem	You generally like yourself and have a good self-esteem. You think generally positively of others while realising that you and they have faults. You are able to trust others, and make a commitment in relationships. This is a healthy state to be in and to aim for	☐
Developing a low sense of worth/self-esteem You doubt whether you can be loved. You may believe you are unattractive, boring or unlovable. There may be all sorts of fears that if others knew the 'real' you they would run a mile	You put on a front and can't be yourself. You can end up being clingy and dependent in relationships and passively do anything to keep a partner happy. You may use alcohol or drugs because you think they make you more 'interesting'	☐
Developing the opposite of the above – a high but fragile self-esteem You may have been taught as a child that you can do anything, that the whole world revolves around you. You see yourself as special. If there are problems, these are caused by others not you	You can be very demanding of others. Things must revolve around you. You need to get your own way. You are often impatient with others who don't 'see the point'. You may seek out passive partners who will look up to you and do what you want. At the same time you may know you could always do better. Job titles and roles really matter. Yet you may quickly feel dissatisfied with jobs and people and want to move on	☐

What you may have learnt from past experience	How this affects your relationships now (your relationship style)	Tick here if this applies to you – even if only sometimes
Thinking of yourself as ugly, unattractive or unlovable	You may feel uncomfortable and avoid close relationships and commitment to protect yourself from hurt ('It will never last'). You are uncomfortable being touched intimately by others. You may dress down and cover up any attractive features by wearing looser clothes. You may give up and let yourself 'go'. Alternatively you may become obsessed that you must look 'just right'. You may flirt or sleep around to test whether you are really attractive, or you may constantly test the love of those who care about you	☐
Others are untrustworthy You may have learned that people you love let you down or abandon you	You may find it difficult to commit or respond with trust to others – even when they want to make a commitment to you. Your lack of trust may end up driving them away	☐
Sometimes your doubts can lead to jealous worries or anger	Jealousy comes from fear and can severely damage your relationships. You may make demands that your partner never goes out alone, especially with other women. You may accuse them of being attracted to others, or become obsessed with pampering and pleasing them in clingy ways that suffocate and restrict	☐

What you may have learnt from past experience	How this affects your relationships now (your relationship style)	Tick here if this applies to you – even if only sometimes
That others use you sexually You may have learned that sex is something to just do, or have done to you. You may have been taught that sex is dirty or wrong, or it is about power/winning and getting your own way	You may withdraw from the possibility of sex. You cannot enjoy this aspect of life or use sex to get what you want. These rules may prevent you from developing a sex life where you can have trust, commitment and enjoyment. Sometimes you may end up in patterns of relationship with partners who make demands and do not respect you	☐
Not showing your emotions You may have learned it's dangerous to show your emotions, or that being seen to be upset is a sign of weakness	The stereotype is that men bottle up their emotions. They use drink or work to block how they feel. Women may be happier discussing their emotions and relationships with others. Of course both patterns can occur with either gender. What matters more is the match (or **mismatch**) between two people For example, when one partner feels distressed and is struggling to cope, they may desperately want to discuss issues in the relationship/life etc. but their partner may not want or feel able to. This clash of styles can lead to further difficulties	☐

Repeating patterns in relationships

The rules you have just read about explain why sometimes you repeat the same patterns in relationships over and over again. They can help you understand why people always go for the same type of person and why they sometimes keep making the same mistakes. Being aware of these patterns is the first step towards changing them.

Key point

You **can** learn new rules.

It's important to be aware of the rules and beliefs you have about you, your family, friends and relatives. They will affect what sorts of styles/patterns of relating you have in relationships.

Partners come second

Having a baby changes your life. But you probably didn't need anyone to tell you that! One thing that many men aren't prepared for is how they can inadvertently often feel squeezed out of being the focus of attention by their baby. Biologically and socially, there is a need for the baby to come first. Some men take to this very well, others can feel threatened. Some go into a sulk or throw a tantrum. If you are feeling down anyway, and especially if you feel you are struggling, the last thing you need right now is a partner or spouse who is feeling touchy.

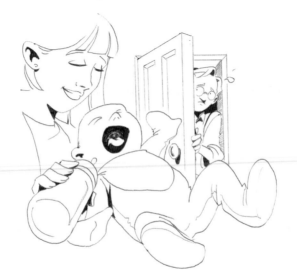

You'll read later how if someone is feeling they are being ignored more than usual they can come to feel very sensitive about things. So if, for example, you don't feel like having sex (because of a tear while giving birth, or tiredness, or loss of interest because of depression – or just because you don't fancy it), your partner may think that things are on the rocks and they are being rejected. There's more on this later, but first think some more about how you relate to important others around us.

How do you relate to others you are close to?

The following questions will help you to recognise your own attitudes and reactions towards others you are close to, such as your partner, spouse, parent or other children. It may be tempting to answer these questions quite quickly with what you think as the 'correct' answer. You'll get the most from this though if you really think about the questions. The purpose is to help you to begin to think about things that may need to change for you to build more balanced relationships.

How do I respond to people I get close to – and how do they respond to me?

Think back on your current and past close relationships.

Q What *helpful* relationship styles do you repeat? (Things you do that build closeness and respect).

Q What *unhelpful* relationship styles do you repeat? (Things you do that damage closeness and reduce respect).

Q How do these patterns affect your relationships – now and in the past?

Q How might these factors affect how you respond when you feel distressed?

Q Do you often feel uncomfortable when speaking about how you or someone close to you feels?

Q Do you try to avoid speaking about how you feel? How do those around you react to this?

Key point

Unhelpful patterns may not affect you for much of the time. However, they can come to the surface when you're feeling more distressed. They then affect how you react to those around you.

What factors have shaped my attitudes and responses?

Think about the things from the past (your upbringing, childhood memories and comments that your parents, friends, others you respect or people from popular culture have made) that affect how you approach intimate relationships.

 How has your own upbringing affected your view of how to relate to those you are close to?

Things you can do that can make a difference

The following are some things you can do (and not do) to build relationships.

With people you don't know so well (like neighbours or people you meet)

Do:

- Be yourself.

- Have planned a brief one-line statement of how you are if someone asks 'How are you?'. Remember, they don't know you well. They may well not be aware you are finding things difficult at the moment. Don't feel you have to tell the person everything about yourself. Say something like 'Getting on fine thanks. How are you? Great weather isn't it?' and leave it at that.

Don't:

- Tell everyone about every aspect of your life and how you feel – this is something you do with a therapist, other health worker or trusted friend.

With trusted friends and family members

Your wider family and friends can be a great support for you. A separate workbook *Information for families and friends – how can you offer the best support?* has been written for them. You might wish to show that workbook to them or even go through it together.

Do

- Seek out support from close friends.

Don't

- Push people away and try to cope by yourself when you need help.

- Become overly focused on just one friendship or just on your baby.

- Confuse friendship and sex. Don't damage a good confiding friendship by something that 'just happened'.

With your partner/husband/boyfriend

Your partner/husband/boyfriend may be your closest support and companion so this relationship can have a big effect on how you feel. Sometimes difficulties may arise and there may be anger, jealousy, boredom, break-ups and affairs. These problems often are the result of a breakdown of communication and even love.

- **Communication**. Communication problems can happen in any relationship, but it becomes even more difficult when you are low or stressed. Having a baby can be a good opportunity to talk more (about how they are, sharing tasks and work, etc.). But sometimes the tasks take over and it's hard to think of anything else than survival. You may not feel like talking, or hugs, or lack the energy or motivation to talk for long. Sometimes these changes are sudden, but more often they slowly build up over the months and years. After a while you may find you have nothing to say. You may find that you do not even know how to even start a conversation. Your partner feels like a stranger.

- **Sex**. You may lose interest in sex, or become anxious about whether you are still as attractive after having the baby. Breastfeeding may change how you feel about sex.

- **The internet**. You may develop a sense of emotional closeness with someone you have never met by chatting with them online. But be careful that this doesn't replace the closeness and support that people around you can offer.

- **Affairs**. Sometimes people try to jolt themselves out of low mood by having a one-night stand or starting an affair. Sometimes this is caused by loneliness, low self-esteem or anger. Some people may look at pornographic pictures or use telephone sex lines or dating agencies that promise 'discreet' relationships. Your partner may have reacted similarly.

- **Time apart**. A symptom of a relationship in trouble is often that we make choices not to be around each other as much. Do you make excuses to be elsewhere? Do you or your partner choose to work late, or go out more? Sometimes people cope by throwing themselves into looking after their children. Children may provide the sense of emotional connection that is missing in their marriage/relationship. People can drift apart even when they are in the same room. For example, never really talking while watching television.

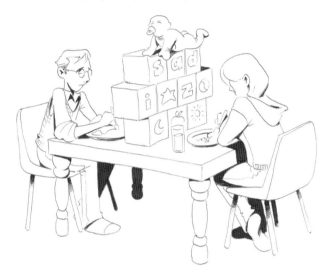

Ultimately these problems come down to the issues of **communication** and **commitment**.

Rebuilding relationships by building communication and commitment

A key question is how much improvement you both feel you need to make to improve things. To rebuild (or build) a relationship can sometimes come down to one partner making all the changes. But that misses the point of the need for *both* partners to discuss and work on their relationship problems together.

It may be that only some small changes of direction are needed. If so, some immediate things you can do together include:

- Listening. Pay attention – don't just switch off and think you know what is being said. Talk about each other's day. Ask questions about the small but important details in life.

- Doing things together – for example, spending time walking the baby or eating meals together as a family rather than separately.

- Tackling 'relationship killers' such as doing things apart.

- Anger and guilt can eat away at a relationship – you may need to forgive your partner – or ask for forgiveness from them if you have done things that have caused hurt.

- Developing physical intimacy in your everyday life at a level that you both feel happy with. Hugs, kisses and holding hands can build bridges. If you don't feel like having sex, try to discuss this. Be clear that it isn't that you don't find your partner attractive or care for them. Try to agree that although you may not want to have sex as often (or even at all at the moment), you still like hugs/kisses. Remember that even though you aren't interested in sex at the moment, your partner still has their sexual needs. Experiment and find activities that will satisfy both you and your partner's sexual needs.

- Bringing back the romance – giving surprises like a small gift, and compliments, or cooking a nice meal. It's the thought and preparation time that matters here – not the cost. Extravagant gifts are no replacement for time together.

Hearing what we expect to hear

At the heart of many relationship problems is a lack of communication. When people have drifted apart there is likely to be blame on both sides and people feel hurt. When someone is distressed they tend to interpret things in quite extreme and unhelpful ways. This can strongly affect how two people interpret the same conversation.

People often think they know each other so well that **they think they already know what is going to be said**. So they don't actually listen to what is being said. The trouble is that sometimes they can be wrong.

> ### Example: Are you hearing what you expect to hear or are you listening to what is being said?
>
> One partner may say something like 'That was a nice meal' and mean this as a compliment. However, because of suspicion and upset, their partner may hear it as 'Well you've cooked something nice for once – usually you don't make much effort'.
>
> Sometimes people can be sarcastic when they offer compliments, but the danger is interpreting all sorts of positive or neutral replies in a negative way.
>
> Likewise, don't assume that others around you can read your mind. Sometimes you may not say what you want and then feel upset when people don't act as you want them to!

📌 Task

Try this test to see if you both interpret the same event in the same way. Think about a time when you have both felt hurt, angry or upset. Then do this exercise when the heat has gone out of the episode. First both of you should separately complete the thought worksheet at the end of this workbook. When you have done this, compare what you have both written by answering the following questions:

How did the same situation affect how you both felt and what you did?

- Do you both agree on exactly what happened?

- If there is a difference in how you both see things?

- Can this help explain your reactions?

- Could this sort of different perception be happening again and again?

What to do if this is an issue

First, identify it as a problem. You can do this by deciding that in future arguments/upsets you will both take stock and choose to clarify and check out what the other is saying. This will help you to avoid jumping to conclusions about each other. Don't do this in an accusatory way – but simply agree that if either of you isn't quite sure of what the other really means you will ask. Ask politely and not in an angry or defensive way.

Try to rein in any immediate reactions if you feel upset, angry or hurt and instead **check it out**. If the other person is trying to be critical this will quickly come out, but often you may find that you've both got the wrong end of the stick.

Some difficult issues

If your partner **feels like a total stranger** to you and you want to rebuild things, you both need to go back to the basics. Be open and discuss how you feel. Jointly decide what you want to do about things. If you both want to tackle this then agree some ground rules about things such as time together, sharing the household tasks and child care responsibilities, eating together and sex. Slowly it is possible to rebuild a sense of love. Expect things to be difficult for some time as you both try to make the changes needed.

Sometimes there may have been an affair, or awful things done or said. Things may have got so bad for other reasons that **someone may have moved out**.

There may be a lot of emotional hurt around. Again you both need to be open and discuss how you feel, and what you want to do about this. Can things recover – or is it too late? These are times of very great challenges in the relationship to you both. Also because there is at least one child or more around, things are even more complicated.

Sometimes relationships end at this stage in recrimination and anger – or just a sense of sadness. Sometimes they can move to that of friendship. Often things can still be rebuilt. Time can heal things. Counselling such as through Relate (see end of workbook) can help even very late in the day, but both people need to want to change things. You can also meet or phone a Relate counsellor in person by yourself or as a couple to help you decide what you want to do.

Violence and threats of violence

If there is violence towards you or anyone else in the family then you need to be clear this is unacceptable. **If you or your child/children are being threatened or hit** you should think about leaving home – or ask your partner to leave at least for a time. Men can sometimes be abused too and may feel shame and isolation. Any violence or aggression is unacceptable. You need to make sure that children are protected.

Many people feel powerless and stuck in violent relationships – or too scared to leave. If you are in this situation you should seek professional help, for example talking to your doctor, or contacting social services or the police. If you are scared to contact these services, talk things through with a trusted friend and go with them. One thing you can be certain about is that unless things change your relationship will end up being destroyed one way or another. The phonebook often gives the number of **local domestic violence helplines** and support agencies. These are confidential and can be a good source of advice. The National Domestic Violence Helpline is 0808 2000 247 or you can check out this website: **www.womensaid.org.uk**

If you yourself are hitting/harming your partner or children then you need to recognise that this is unacceptable. Sometimes this may be new behaviour you have developed as a result of anger linked to your depression or tension. Sometimes it's an effect of drink. Violence and threats may be something that you have done for a long time and in a variety of relationships. Either way, it's important that you recognise that you are hurting the people whom you love and must stop. Look for times when you are prone to losing control (for example when you drink) and tackle this. You may find it helpful to join an anger management group. Your doctor or health visitor can give you more information about this. Reducing how much you drink can help and so can getting treatment for any depression or anxiety. You will feel better for it – and you may be able to save and rebuild your relationship too.

Sometimes the extent of the relationship breakdown may be that you need professional advice such as counselling. Charities such as Relate can help with this.

Key point

Ultimately, although many relationships can be rebuilt or lived with, sometimes they can't, and a time apart or permanent separation may result.

To find your nearest Relate centre call Relate General Enquiries on 0845 456 1310 (local rate applies). For a telephone counselling appointment call 0845 130 4016.

 www.relate.org.uk

Summary

In this workbook you have:

- Reviewed your own style of communicating with others.

- Learnt how to play, enjoy and build a loving relationship with your baby.

- Learnt how to build (and rebuild close) relationships with the people around you.

- Found out how to develop a new identity as a mother which includes your old friends.

Putting into practice what you have learned

Re-read what you learned earlier in the *Being assertive* workbook about the 'broken record' and 'saying no' approaches, and try to practise using them during the next week. In particular, the 'saying no' approach allows you to plan out how to be assertive in a particular situation and with a specific person. View this as a sort of action plan that can help you to both change how you are, and also learn something new about yourself and other people.

If anger or low confidence are major problems for you, you can try to read these two short books dealing with these problems:

● *Are You Strong Enough to Keep Your Temper?* by Chris Williams.

● *I'm Not Good Enough: How to Overcome Low Confidence* by Chris Williams.

 You can buy these books from our website (**www.fiveareas.com**).

If relationships are a problem for you, consider showing this workbook to your partner. Read it through together. You might also want to go through the *Information for families and friends – how can you offer the best support?* workbook as well.

My notes

My Five Areas thought review of a time when I felt worse

Write down your feelings and thoughts in all five areas of your life:

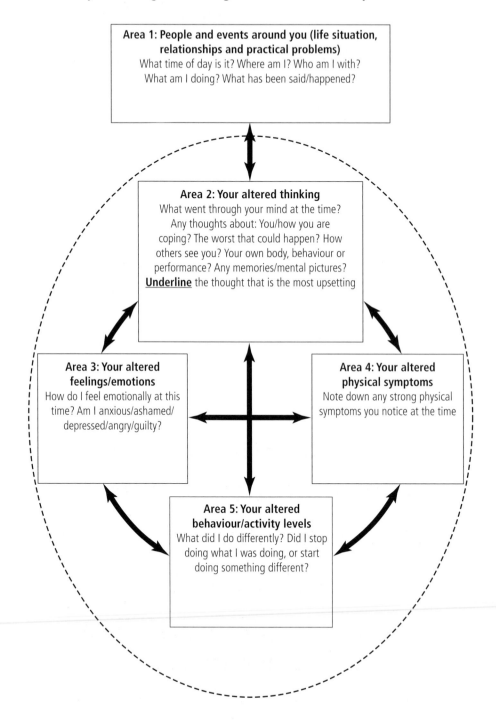

Area 1: People and events around you (life situation, relationships and practical problems)
What time of day is it? Where am I? Who am I with? What am I doing? What has been said/happened?

Area 2: Your altered thinking
What went through your mind at the time? Any thoughts about: You/how you are coping? The worst that could happen? How others see you? Your own body, behaviour or performance? Any memories/mental pictures? **Underline** the thought that is the most upsetting

Area 3: Your altered feelings/emotions
How do I feel emotionally at this time? Am I anxious/ashamed/depressed/angry/guilty?

Area 4: Your altered physical symptoms
Note down any strong physical symptoms you notice at the time

Area 5: Your altered behaviour/activity levels
What did I do differently? Did I stop doing what I was doing, or start doing something different?

Overcoming Postnatal Depression
A Five Areas Approach

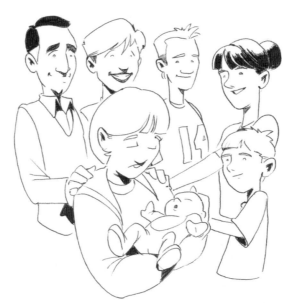

Information for families and friends – how can you offer the best support?

www.livinglifetothefull.com
www.fiveareas.com

Dr Chris Williams, Dr Roch Cantwell and
Karen Robertson

I'm really worried about her

You're suffocating me

She's always saying she doesn't want to talk

I don't know what to say

She's so frustrating!

I must make her see sense

We must do everything for her

I feel like I'm walking on eggshells

Are you feeling like this?

If so … this workbook is for you.

This workbook is for the family and friends of mothers who are feeling unwell with postnatal depression. It also tells you more about the 'Overcoming postnatal depression' course so that family and friends can understand and offer support in the best possible way.

In this workbook you will learn about:

- What this course is about – and how the person is using it.

- How best to help and communicate effectively.

- Helpful things you can do so that you can offer the support that the person needs.

- Unhelpful things that you should try not to do, which can undermine the support you can give.

- Looking after yourself as a friend or relative so that you stay well.

- Putting what you've learnt into practice.

Background for friends and family

The course workbooks use a proved approach based on cognitive behaviour therapy (CBT, a kind of talking treatment). CBT is a treatment that's known to work well for people who are facing many problems in their life – including stress and low mood. An important part of your role is to provide support – and also an objective viewpoint. This can help encourage the person and keep them on track while they try to work on their problems.

The approach used in the course looks in detail at five important areas of life. The **Five Areas assessment** helps a person recognise the kinds of problems they may be facing in each of the following areas:

1. The people and events around them (their situation).

2. Their thinking (with extreme and unhelpful thinking).

3. Their feelings (emotions).

4. Their altered bodily sensations (their physical symptoms).

5. Their behaviour (any altered behaviour or activity levels).

Key point

What we think about a situation or problem may affect how we feel emotionally and physically. It can also alter what we do.

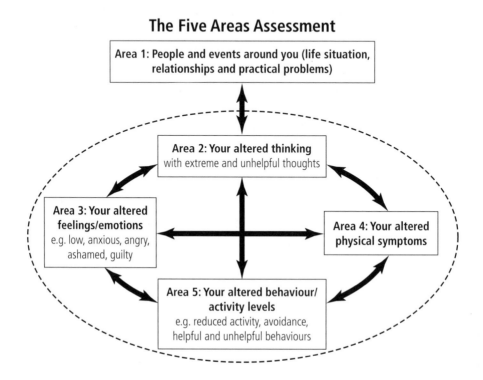

The Five Areas Assessment

Area 1: People and events around you (life situation, relationships and practical problems)

Area 2: Your altered thinking
with extreme and unhelpful thoughts

Area 3: Your altered feelings/emotions
e.g. low, anxious, angry, ashamed, guilty

Area 4: Your altered physical symptoms

Area 5: Your altered behaviour/activity levels
e.g. reduced activity, avoidance, helpful and unhelpful behaviours

Because of the links between each of the five areas, the actions that people take can worsen or keep their symptoms going. Importantly, it also means that helpful changes in any one of the areas can lead to benefits in the others areas as well. Finally, it means that **the people around the person can also help change things**.

About the workbook approach

The course workbooks aim to help mothers by:

- Giving them useful information about how postnatal depression is affecting their life.

- Teaching them important life skills to help make useful changes in the five areas of their life.

They are practical workbooks, which means the person has to stop, think and reflect on the impact their symptoms can have on their life.

The workbooks are usually used by the person on their own. They are used one at a time – and the reader is encouraged to read them slowly. This allows them to practise what they have learned over a week or so before moving on to the next one. The person can discuss the workbooks (if she wants) with others, such as family members, friends or a healthcare practitioner. Each workbook is their own resource and is private to them. Some mothers find it helpful to share them – but you need to respect their wishes here. The workbooks are like someone's personal diary and in the same way they aren't meant to be read by everyone.

However, this particular workbook is designed to be read and discussed jointly.

How can you help?

One of the most important things is to encourage the person to use the workbooks. Probably the best two words to describe this are **supportive encouragement**. Support means:

● Being interested.

● Being hopeful.

● Encouraging the person to try things out – give it a go.

● Suggesting or freeing up a time when they can use the materials, for example, you can help by looking after the baby and any other children for an hour or so.

● Encouraging not badgering.

● Asking how you can help – some people prefer to work alone or with someone independent such as their health worker.

It's important to remember that you are the friend or relative and not the therapist. Let the workbooks do the teaching and the therapeutic work. Your role is to help the person understand and work them into action in their own life.

Other ways of supporting – keeping talking

A common problem that happens when someone is struggling is that their family or friends may not fully understand what is happening or know how to offer help. This is because you may have never experienced what the person is going through yourself. When this happens, it can lead to further problems such as frustration and withdrawal.

Sometimes the person who is unwell can become preoccupied with how she feels and she struggles to communicate. Seeing each other's point of view at times like this is important. The danger is when either party starts to think that those around them no longer care. Stating clearly what you are thinking and feeling here can really help move things forward.

You may have all sorts of other worries. You may be concerned about the reactions of other people to your friend's or relative's problem. For example, the attitude and comments of neighbours, colleagues, bosses, healthcare practitioners, people at your place of worship and other friends or relatives. It could be you think that you don't know how to respond or offer support beyond the short term, such as giving flowers and 'Get well' cards. Or when you've tried to help, you were uncertain how best to do this. You may struggle to know what to say. If you feel like this you may be tempted to avoid talking about the person's symptoms as a result.

If you feel that you can't talk through how things are – or are unsure how either of you can show that you care – then this workbook is for you.

Understanding the causes of postnatal depression

When a person breaks their leg, there is a large plaster cast on the leg to see. Similarly if you have a chest infection there is lots of green phlegm to cough into tissues. In people with cancer, some cells in their body grow too quickly and in those with heart disease, blocked blood vessels cause them the pain called angina. Physical illnesses such as these are very visible or can be picked up on scans of the body. But some symptoms aren't so visible, for example problems of tiredness, weakness, dizziness and pain. The same is true of feelings of sadness, stress and tension which again are not visible in the same way as a broken leg, heart disease or cancer.

Some relatives and friends find they just can't understand how someone can become depressed. They see, for example, the happiness of a new baby and think that there's no reason why depression should occur. But remember that depression can strike anyone at any time. In many ways, postnatal depression is the same as depression that occurs at any other stage in life. There are lots of different factors – physical, psychological, social – that affect whether a person gets depression. Even 'happy' events like Christmas can be a cause of depression. Similarly, the challenges and stresses of having a baby may start off a low mood.

The important thing is that whatever the cause of your friend or relative's depression, you are there to help.

How to offer help

Now complete the following checklist. It will help you recognise your friend or relative's strengths and possible problems that you may wish to tackle together. You might find it helpful to first go through the checklist separately and then discuss your answers to each question together.

Q Can you identify some common problems that can arise for the sufferer?

- Isolation: your friend or relative finds it hard to talk to and receive support from others.

  Yes ☐   No ☐   Sometimes ☐

- There is just no-one around who they can really talk to.

  Yes ☐   No ☐   Sometimes ☐

- You or others are unsure how to best offer support.

  Yes ☐   No ☐   Sometimes ☐

- You or others have begun to drop away from offering support.

  Yes ☐   No ☐   Sometimes ☐

- You or others are avoiding talking about your friend or relative's symptoms and their impact.

  Yes ☐   No ☐   Sometimes ☐

- Perhaps even their healthcare practitioners may struggle to offer the kind of support needed.

Yes ☐　　　　　No ☐　　　　　Sometimes ☐

- Are the symptoms not 'visible' or obvious to others?

Yes ☐　　　　　No ☐　　　　　Sometimes ☐

- If 'Yes': does this seem to affect how others react?

Yes ☐　　　　　No ☐　　　　　Sometimes ☐

Write down what you have both noticed here:

Avoiding things

When people feel anxious or worried about things, they often avoid situations, other people, places, or even conversations that they feel may be difficult or stressful. This adds to their problems because although they may feel less anxious or unwell in the shorter term, in the longer term such actions can worsen the problem.

Key point

The problem with avoidance is that it teaches you that the only way of dealing with a difficult situation is by avoiding it. The avoidance reduces your opportunities to find out that your worst fears don't occur. It worsens anxiety and strongly undermines your confidence.

Example: John and Sally's vicious circles of avoidance

John's partner Sally gave birth to their baby, Jack, eight weeks ago. Since then Sally has felt increasingly low in mood. Her confidence has taken a huge knock and she is finding she can no longer cope with things. She tends to sit indoors – crying from time to time about things she hasn't done around the house.

A real issue for Sally is that she feels embarrassed when things aren't neat and clean. Sally is very uneasy that John is getting annoyed at her for letting things pile up. She feels deeply ashamed of how things are and is very upset.

John is also concerned about Sally. He knows that she isn't herself. He expected them both to be tired (and they certainly are) but now the 'spark' seems to have gone out of Sally, and she seems really ground down by her symptoms. The health visitor has been checking up on Sally and has told John that she has postnatal depression, and there is talk about taking anti-depressant tablets.

John wants to speak to Sally about how worried he is – and how he wants to help. As a person though, he has always struggled to be open about how he feels – and Sally isn't much different. Although they know they love each other they both find it hard to talk about the depression.

Now John sits thinking 'We *should be discussing things – how can I help?*'. He has tried to bring up his concerns and suggested they get a cleaner, but Sally quickly becomes defensive and seems embarrassed.

Both Sally and John think: 'What can we do?'

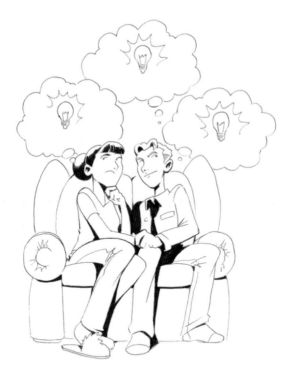

Q How are Sally and John's reactions worsening the situation?

Q What could they do to change things?

Sometimes, even *talking about the symptoms* can become a topic that is avoided at home or with friends. Even among close relatives and friends there may be an embarrassment over discussing things.

 Task

The checklist below describes common areas of avoidance.

Family and friends checklist: Identifying the vicious circle of avoidance

As a friend/family member, are you:	Tick here if you have noticed this – even if just sometimes
Completely avoiding asking about anything to do with postnatal depression?	☐
Avoiding talking to anyone else about your friend or relative's symptoms or about how they are coping?	☐
Putting off all decisions until the person is better. For example, putting holidays or other life plans completely on hold	☐
Not really being honest with others or with your friend or relative. For example, saying 'Yes' when you really mean 'No'?	☐
Trying hard to avoid situations that bring about upsetting thoughts/memories?	☐
Brooding over things and therefore no longer living your own life to the full?	☐
Avoiding discussing how you yourself are feeling or coping?	☐
Avoiding people/isolating yourself from others?	☐
Avoiding expressing concerns about how the baby is doing if there is a clear problem here? If there is, it's important to make sure the care that is needed is given. Discussing these concerns with a professional is important.	☐
Avoiding being assertive about your own needs?	☐

© Dr Chris Williams (2009)

As a friend/family member, are you:	Tick here if you have noticed this – even if just sometimes
Avoiding going out in public either by yourself or with the person you are supporting?	☐
Avoiding being at home: keeping so busy that you don't have to think about the problem?	☐
For partners/spouses:	
Avoiding sex or physical intimacy? Perhaps there may be fears of over-exertion or causing harm? Or issues about whether this would be imposing/inappropriate or not wanted at present?	☐

Q Are you avoiding things in other ways?

Write down here how you are doing this if this is so:

Sometimes, some of these questions can be hard to discuss. This may especially be so around issues such as sex or intimacy. You can always decide to discuss them at a later time but don't ignore them as they are important.

Remember that at times the avoidance can be quite subtle. For example, choosing to steer conversations away from difficult areas that would actually benefit from being discussed. Often people fear upsetting the other person or making them feel worse. This can backfire, however, because it means issues aren't dealt with and certain topics can keep building up as things that 'must not be discussed'.

Overcoming avoidance with clear communication

The only way of overcoming avoidance is openness and honesty. Without this many problems can arise. If you are someone who worries about hurting other people's feelings, or aren't quite sure how to discuss these things openly, then you might find the *Being assertive* and *Building relationships with your baby, family and friends* workbooks helpful.

Building relationships

Here are some practical phrases and strategies you can use to relate differently to each other.

- 'This isn't a good time to talk, let's talk about it later.'
- Sometimes people need to work through an issue by talking at length. Let them talk, often no comment is needed. Listen for the main message, and then pick up on this point so the person knows you are really listening. For example 'It sounds like you feel frustrated/fed up today ...'
- Offer praise and encouragement to build confidence, for example 'I can see such a difference from a month or so ago ...'
- Actively look for things you can comment positively about.
- Try to find at least three positive things to say every day.

Mother, baby and you: getting the right balance

It can be hard to know how much help to offer with a new baby. Mothers with postnatal depression struggle to cope with their symptoms and also their babies. It can be tempting to offer practical help with the baby care. This is quite understandable and helpful, but again this is an issue of balance.

Women with postnatal depression often feel they have failed as a mother. Having someone step in and apparently take over runs the risk of undermining their confidence. Support should therefore be shared as much as possible ('Can I help you so we can change his nappy together ...').

Also try to encourage play time between the mother and her baby. A common view held by mothers when they are depressed is that everyone else is lots more fun for the baby than they are and that the baby responds more to others than to them. They often worry that they and their depression may be harming the development of their baby. Again, often a helpful approach is to arrange joint play where you, the mother/parents and baby can all sit on the playmat and take turns. In this way you will help to build up the relationship between mother and baby. There are also lots of opportunities during the day to point out how their relationship is developing ('Look at how she smiles at you as you gave her that cuddle').

Helpful and unhelpful responses

When someone you care about needs your help you try to improve things through different actions. Mostly, your actions are *helpful* responses that can improve how they and you feel. Sometimes however – without meaning to – how you react can become *unhelpful*.

This section focuses on both the helpful and possible unhelpful behaviours that friends/relatives/carers may do.

Helpful activities by family and friends

- Finding out about postnatal depression, for example, by reading the workbooks in this course or other information booklets, getting information from self-help groups or from healthcare practitioners. This can equip you with the knowledge and skills you need. You may find looking at the online course at **www.livinglifetothefull.com** helpful. (This is an added resource to support users of this workbook).

- 'Being there' for the person for the long term.

- Being willing to talk and offer support when needed.

- Encouraging asking questions of experts such as the health visitor.

- Encouraging the person to put what they are learning in this course into practice.

- Keeping a positive but realistic outlook that change is possible but will take time.

- Realising there are no quick fixes.

- Using your sense of humour to help you and the person you support to cope.

- Planning time for yourself as well as for others.

- Using effective coping responses, such as relaxation techniques, to deal with your feelings of tension.

- Looking after yourself.

- Seeing a healthcare practitioner for advice if you yourself are struggling to cope.

- Pacing recovery. Recovering from depression takes time. Even when mood improves, there is a period of weeks to months where a person is more vulnerable to relapse. Think about the broken leg again. When the plaster comes off, you wouldn't expect to run a marathon the next day! Muscles need to be built up again. In the same way, although the depression may lift, a person needs to build up their confidence and activities slowly again. Helping them pace their recovery is one of the best ways of reducing the risk of relapse.

Q Are you doing anything else that is helpful?

Unhelpful behaviours by family and friends

Sometimes family and friends can think that something they are doing is helpful when in fact it's part of the problem. For example, wrapping the person in cotton wool, taking over everything from them, or bullying and forcing them to do something. Sometimes people can also react out of frustration to 'let off steam'. Although this can make you feel better initially this can also backfire and create further problems. For example, some people may find that raising their voice in frustration can make them feel a lot better to begin with. But this can have a damaging effect on your relationship and leave you feeling guilty.

Key point

The hallmark of a truly helpful activity is that it's good for you and often for others as well.

One way of thinking about this is that no matter how helpful something may seem to begin with, if taken to an extreme most responses can backfire. For example, seeking support from others is sensible. A problem shared can really help – but if you find that your friend or relative is constantly on the phone and feels she can't cope without talking to others to reassure her then again something that was originally helping has become a problem.

Other unhelpful behaviours include:

- Offering 'helpful advice' **all the time**.

- A desire to do **everything** for the person.

- **Constantly** offering reassurance that everything will work out fine ('Of course you'll be okay').

- Overly protecting and suffocating the person by taking away **all** their responsibility (and all their choices too).

You can see that the words in bold here make this same point again. The motive may be good, and some of these actions may be helpful to some extent. But when taken to excess, they become unhelpful.

There are many reasons why people behave in this way. Often it's due to concern, friendship and love. Sometimes it may be the result of anxiety, or occasionally guilt. Whatever the cause, when people offer too much help and want to do everything for someone else, their actions can backfire and worsen things.

Frustration and anger at healthcare practitioners

It isn't unusual that when someone takes on a supportive or carer role they can struggle themselves. Different feelings such as demoralisation, worry, guilt, frustration or even anger can occur. These frustrations can spill over into how you talk about healthcare practitioners.

It can be tempting to become critical. Most healthcare practitioners can offer helpful support to people. But from time to time, even those working in the caring professions may not be able to offer the kind of support that you feel your friend or relative needs.

Key point

If you are too critical of healthcare practitioners, there is a danger that you will undermine the support and advice that they can offer.

But what if you disagree?

Sometimes people have strong opinions about what treatments or investigations the friend or relative whom they are supporting may need. For example, a person may have strong opinions about alternative and complementary medicine approaches or just not be happy that the current treatment is working. They may have understandable worries about medication during pregnancy or breastfeeding.

If your friend or relative is being offered treatments or investigations that you have concerns about, it's important to be aware of how you respond. If they have been prescribed medication try not to persuade them to suddenly stop taking their medication without discussing it with their doctor. If you have strong concerns that a treatment is wrong or not needed it is best for you both to go along (if the person who is unwell is happy for this) to the doctor to discuss things. What all of you want is the best possible outcome. This is especially the case when anti-depressants are prescribed, because people would prefer it if the person they are supporting could recover without them. It is important to remember here that postnatal depression is a serious problem and needs treatment in the same way as serious depression does at other times. It's also important for a baby that their mother recovers as quickly as possible. The doctor will have thought about things such as breastfeeding when deciding to prescribe anti-depressants.

Task

Look at the following list of common unhelpful behaviours. Tick any activity you have found yourself doing over the last month.

Family and friends checklist: unhelpful behaviours

As a friend/family member, are you:	Tick here if you have noticed this – even if just sometimes
Becoming overly protective of the person – wrapping them in cotton wool?	☐
Taking overall responsibility from the person? For example, making all the important decisions, with no discussion, or trying to control every aspect of their life. (The result is undermined confidence and often resentment)	☐
Taking over all activities they used to do so they do not have to 'worry' about them? For example, things they used to enjoy or be responsible for, such as household tasks, taking children to school, feeling the need to earn more so they do not have to work	☐
Not allowing the person to be upset or distressed? For example, trying to 'buck them up' all the time	☐
Having a go at the person from time to time – through frustration or anger?	☐
Becoming so focused on the distressed person that other people's needs aren't met? For example, your own or other family members such as children are overlooked	☐
Depending on or needing the sufferer to be well and functioning? (So that they aren't allowed to be unwell)	☐
Talking only about how hard things are? This contributes to a downward emotional spiral	☐
Making snap decisions about important issues? For example, resigning a post	☐
Automatically advising the person not to try certain treatment approaches because of your fears that it may do harm?	☐
Undermining or criticising healthcare practitioners? (Because they haven't been able to find a cure)	☐
Ignoring or leaving tensions that should be dealt with but are being overlooked because of the focus on caring?	☐

As a friend/family member, are you:	Tick here if you have noticed this – even if just sometimes
Helping the person avoid doing things because of fears about what harm might result? For example, taking over going to the shops, driving. This then further undermines their confidence	☐
Constantly reassuring the person to allay their anxious fears?	☐
Constantly asking how they are? (Which unhelpfully draws attention to illness)	☐
Introducing the person as 'X, who has this problem', rather than just by their name? For example, you have started seeing the symptoms not the person	☐
Telling the person to excessively avoid activities because you are concerned about their health – even if the activities are recommended by their healthcare practitioner?	☐
Speaking for/over the person in social settings, or in hospital outpatients, etc.? For example, you tell their story rather than them	☐

Write in any other unhelpful behaviours here:

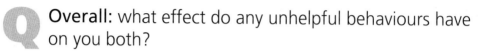

Overall: what effect do any unhelpful behaviours have on you both?

The problem is that these responses can quickly become a habit – where the same pattern is repeated again and again.

Wrapping the person in cotton wool

Offering extra special attention and support can also become unhelpful. The relationship may feel suffocating and frustrating. The person can end up feeling treated like a child. Arguments and little irritations build up and are upsetting all round.

Although in such situations people mean well, your actions can actually undermine your relationship. When your friend or relative is trying to cope with symptoms, it's important to encourage her to keep as active as possible within the confines of how she feels. If you take responsibility for doing everything, the danger is that she will not be as active as she could be and so you create unnecessary dependency.

Faith and seeking help

Parents or other carers may have a strong spiritual belief. This may be very helpful, but sometimes these beliefs can emphasise prayer as the only way towards recovery and healing.

People can tend to ignore that health workers may have an important part in the recovery process, and they may be part of an answer to prayer. In the same way that you would recommend someone seek medical help if they broke their arm or leg, the person needs to seek medical help for low mood and depression. If you have doubts about how medical help can help low mood and depression, please discuss this with a spiritual leader whom you respect.

Staying well yourself

When you support others you also need to look after yourself and allow time and space for your own needs. Depression and stress are very common among carers. The danger is that you are so busy offering support that you have no time for yourself.

Helpful responses to look after yourself include:

- Open discussion of your own stress – for example, with your own doctor or perhaps within a carer support group.
- Taking short breaks/holidays/weekends away with others.
- Planning 'me time' such as hobbies/interests/night classes into the day and week.
- Attending relaxation or stress management groups/classes or carer support groups.
- Seeing your own doctor to discuss the need for additional treatment and support.

Building helpful behaviours and reducing unhelpful behaviours

To successfully plan a reduction in unhelpful behaviours or to increase helpful behaviours, you need to have a clear plan.

Do:

- Think of a plan to slowly alter what you do in a step-by-step way.
- Plan to alter only one response you make over the next week.
- Make changes one step at a time until you reach your eventual goal.
- Write down your plan in detail so that you will be able to put it into practice this week.

Don't:

- Choose something that is too big a target to start with.
- Try to start to alter too many things all at once.
- Be very negative and think 'Nothing can be done, what's the point, it's a waste of time.' Try to experiment to find out if this negative thinking is accurate or helpful.

The seven-step plan to building helpful behaviours

The seven-step plan described here can help you to plan to do things differently.

Think about how you can begin to tackle the problems you face in your own life. This may be:

- To reduce any unhelpful behaviour.

or

- To build up a helpful behaviour.

You will already have an idea of the different activities you are doing from the checklists you have completed in this workbook. In fact, if you try to change everything at once you might find that you can't change anything. The important first step is thinking of the **single** initial target that you can focus on. This is particularly important if you have ticked several boxes in the checklists. You need to decide which **one** area to concentrate on to start with.

Step 1: Identify and clearly define the problem

Write down the problem here:

Q Is this clear and focused?

Yes ☐   No ☐

If you said 'No', rewrite the problem so that it is clear and focused.

Step 2: Think up as many solutions as possible to achieve this initial goal

It may be that the thought of making changes seems daunting or impossible. But there are all sorts of ways to tackle the problems you may face. Likewise, there are many possible ways to build up helpful behaviours. To help you recognise many possible solutions, try to use an approach called **brainstorming**.

When you are brainstorming, you try to think broadly to come up with as many ideas as possible. Then from among them you hope to be able to identify a realistic, practical and achievable solution. The more solutions that you think of, the more likely it is that a good one will emerge. To start with you should include even completely whacky ideas in your list, even if you would never choose them in practice. This is because it can help you to take a flexible approach to the problem.

Here are some useful questions to help you to think up a good first list of solutions:

- What advice would you give a friend who was trying to tackle the same problem? Sometimes it's easier to think of solutions for others than for yourself.

- What ridiculous solutions can you include as well as more sensible ones?

- What helpful ideas would others (for example, family, friends or colleagues at work) suggest?

- How could you look at the solutions facing you differently? For example, what would you have said before your friend or relative was depressed, or what might you say about the situation say in five years' time?

- What approaches have you tried in the past in similar circumstances?

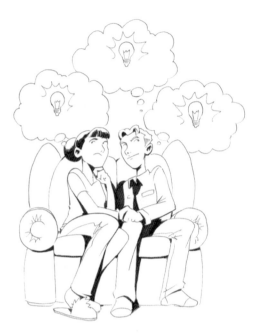

Try to think of as many ideas as you can. If this proves hard, as mentioned above, try to think of some bizarre ones first to help get the ideas flowing.

Brainstorming the problem

Possible ways in which you can help your friend or relative are (including ridiculous ideas at first) are:

Step 3: Look at the pros and cons of each possible solution

Key point

Think of the pros and cons of each solution you have come up with so that you can clearly see which ones are the better ideas.

My suggestions from Step 2	Pros (advantages)	Cons (disadvantages)

Step 4: Now choose one of the solutions

Choose a solution that is a small step in the right direction and you think is more likely to succeed. Base this on all the answers to Step 3.

What you are looking for most often is to find a **step-by-step** approach where no step seems too large. That's why the solution you are looking for is something that gets you moving in the right direction. This should be small enough to be possible, but big enough to move you forwards.

Write down your preferred solution here:

Now check your choice against some of the **Questions for effective change**.

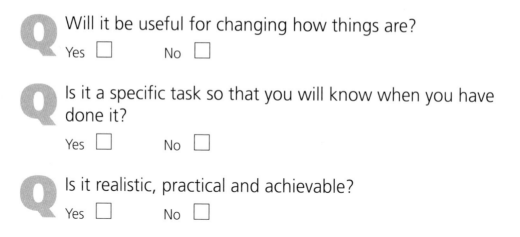

Will it be useful for changing how things are?

Yes ☐   No ☐

Is it a specific task so that you will know when you have done it?

Yes ☐   No ☐

Is it realistic, practical and achievable?

Yes ☐   No ☐

Step 5: Plan the steps needed to carry out your plan

Write down the practical steps needed to carry out your plan. Try to be very specific so that you know *what* you are going to do, and *when* you are going to do it.

Important note: Part of this planning should include planning what you will do if your initial plan doesn't fully work.

Now, write down your plan here:

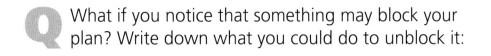 What if you notice that something may block your plan? Write down what you could do to unblock it:

Now check your plan against the rest of the **Questions for effective change**:

Does it make clear what you are going to do and when you are going to do it?

Yes ☐   No ☐

Is it an activity that won't be easily blocked or prevented by practical problems?

Yes ☐   No ☐

Will it help you to learn useful things even if it doesn't work out perfectly?

Yes ☐   No ☐

Step 6: Carry out your plan

Carry out your plan during the next week.

Pay attention to any thoughts and fears about what will happen before, during and after you have completed your plan. Try to do your plan anyway.

Write down any thoughts or fears that you may have noticed:

Step 7: Review the outcome

Write down any helpful lessons or information you have learned from what happened. If things didn't go quite as you hoped, try to learn from this. How could you make things different during your next attempt to try to be helpful?

Q Was your plan successful?

Yes ☐   No ☐

Q Did it help improve things?

Yes ☐   No ☐

Did any problems arise?

Yes ☐   No ☐

Try to learn from any mistakes and keep practising so that using this approach becomes second nature whenever you face a problem or you want to help your friend or relative.

Summary

In this workbook you have learned:

- What this course is about – and how your friend or relative is using it.

- How best to help and communicate effectively.

- Helpful and unhelpful things you can do so that you can offer effective support.

- How to look after yourself and stay well.

What have I learnt from this workbook?

What do I want to try *next*?

Putting what you have learned into practice

Please reflect on the seven-step plan and think how you can use it to:

- Reduce one *unhelpful behaviour* or one area of *avoidance* over the next week.

- Plan to build upon one *helpful response* this week.

Remember: Do not try to do everything all at once. Plan out what to do at a pace that is right for you.

Where to get extra help

Ideally the person with depression has someone like you to support them during their illness. But there are times when this won't be enough. You should support your friend or relative to get extra help if you think they have any of the following:

- **Severe depression**, for example continuing low mood, tearfulness, significant sleep, concentration, weight or energy loss despite attempts to improve things.

- Strong urges to **self-harm** or feeling really **hopeless** or have **suicidal thoughts**.

- Other concerning **dangerous behaviours**, for example risk-taking, threats of harm to others.

- A possibility of immediate or longer-term significant harm or injury by someone else. For example, **abuse or neglect, including concerns for the health or safety of your friend or relative's baby and other children.**

- **Severe withdrawal from life activities**, for example they are clearly not coping well at all.

- **Serious weight loss** or the person has stopped drinking.

There could be other situations as well where extra help is needed or can be a real help and, if in doubt, it's important to ask for help in *deciding* whether more help is needed.

If there is a risk of immediate significant harm (abuse, self-harm or suicide), action will need to be taken immediately. Remember that professional and voluntary services can give a great deal of support.

What if the person doesn't agree they need extra help?

It is always best to get the person's agreement for getting extra help, but sometimes the risks involved may mean help is needed whether they agree or not.

If you are seriously worried that extra help is needed but the person is refusing, then it's still best to ask for help in deciding if anything else should or can be done. Don't just keep it to yourself. If you aren't sure, phone NHS Direct (England and Wales) or NHS 24 (Scotland) (see contact details below). You can discuss the issues through in confidence and will receive sensible advice as to what you should do.

Key point

If you are still worried or concerned, it is better to ask for help or advice than do nothing.

Sources of extra help

- **NHS Direct** for England and Wales (tel: 0845 4647, 24-hour line; website: **www.nhsdirect.nhs.uk**) or **NHS 24** for Scotland (tel: 08454 242424; website: **www.nhs24.nhs.com**).

- Your or the person's doctor or GP.

- **Social services**. You can find your local social services office hours' enquiry phone number and a 24-hour emergency phone number in the *Yellow Pages*.

- **NSPCC**. Adults who are worried about a child can call 0808 800 5000 or visit the NSPCC website (**www.nspcc.org.uk**). The NSPCC has 24-hour helplines (for example NSPCC Child Protection Helpline) that you can call to talk things over without the number appearing on house phone bills.

- Local counselling services, such as **Relate** (see **www.relate.org.uk** or call 0300 100 1234).

- **Royal College of Psychiatrists**. You can get fact sheets about postnatal depression by calling 020 7235 2351 or visiting the college's website (**www.rcpsych.ac.uk/mentalhealthinformation/mentalhealthproblems /postnatalmentalhealth/postnataldepression.aspx**).

You can buy the following helpful books from local or online bookshops or you may find them at your local library:

- *Overcoming Anxiety: A Five Areas Approach* by Dr C Williams.
- *Overcoming Depression and Low Mood: A Five Areas Approach* by Dr C Williams.
- *I'm Not Supposed to Feel Like This: A Christian Self-help Approach to Depression and Anxiety* by Chris Williams, Paul Richards and Ingrid Whitton.
- *Overcoming Low Self-Esteem: A Self-Help Guide to Using Cognitive Behavioural Techniques* by Melanie Fennell.

Short, key skills booklets available from **www.fiveareas.com**:

- Why do I feel so bad?
- How to fix almost everything.
- Why does everything always go wrong?
- I can't be bothered doing anything.
- The things you do that mess you up.
- Are you strong enough to keep your temper (anger).
- I'm not good enough (low confidence).
- 10 things you can do to make you feel happier straight away.
- I feel so bad I can't go on.

… and others

www.livinglifetothefull.com

This is a free online training course that teaches key life skills by using the same model used in this book. The website also provides free access to the online version of the *Living Life to the Full* DVD and more handouts that you can download.

My notes

Overcoming Postnatal Depression
A Five Areas Approach

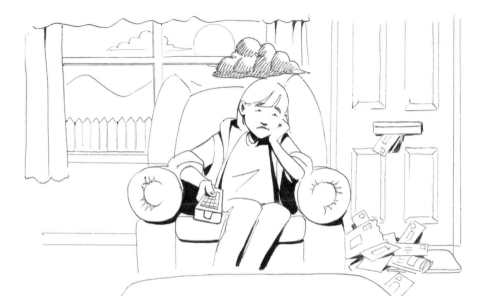

Doing things that boost how you feel

www.livinglifetothefull.com
www.fiveareas.com

Dr Chris Williams, Dr Roch Cantwell and
Karen Robertson

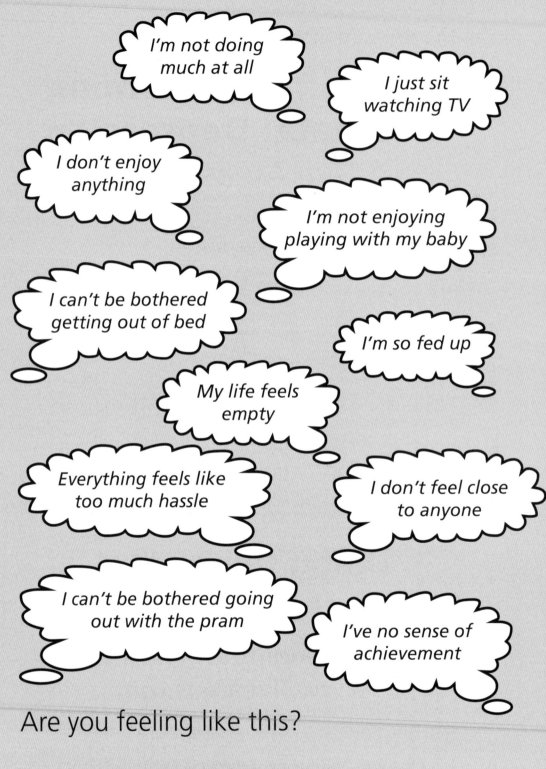

Are you feeling like this?

If so ... this workbook is for you.

In this workbook you will:

- Learn how low mood and stress causes you to do less.

- Find out how reduced activity affects you.

- Record your current activity levels and discover what gives you a boost.

- Plan ways to make slow, steady changes to your life to boost how you feel.

- Plan some next steps to build on these changes.

How low mood can affect you

Having postnatal depression can make life seem much harder. Everything can seem like a struggle. This is because of:

- Low energy and tiredness ('I'm just too tired').

- Low mood – so you don't really enjoy things when you do them.

- Little sense of achievement when things are done – you don't feel any or much satisfaction in a job well done. This makes it seem as if you are on a never-ending treadmill.

- Loss of a sense of closeness to others, for example you might know you want to feel happiness and love for your baby, but you may just feel numb instead.

- Symptoms such as pain, weakness or restricted movement that make getting out a problem. For example, if you had a caesarean or you have on-going problems such as back or pelvic pain. Problems such as these can grind you down and make it harder to keep going as usual.

- Negative thinking and low enthusiasm to do things ('I just can't do it').

The result is that **you struggle to do things and do less and less**. But when you do less, it can make you feel even worse. Have you been so focused on just surviving and doing the essentials that other important things in your life have been squeezed out?

Mothers who have postnatal depression tend to focus on core life activities that '*have*' to be done. This means things such as looking after the baby or other children, doing chores or just struggling by. Other things that you would usually do for fun or friendship slowly just drop away. So, a cycle is set up of feeling low, doing fewer things that lift you, and then feeling worse and worse.

Overcoming Postnatal Depression: A Five Areas Approach   © Dr Chris Williams (2009)

Sometimes mothers also may become so focused on just surviving that you don't have time to sit back and feel a sense of achievement in what you do.

How inactivity can affect you

Doing less changes how you feel emotionally and physically:

- **You feel lower in mood** as described above.

- **You feel physically worse**. When you feel unwell a natural response is to rest. Resting can be helpful, for example to allow a pulled muscle to settle. However, if you rest too much or for too long, your body can show unintended changes, for example your unused muscle will tend to lose muscle bulk and weaken.

In one study, the researchers paid some students to go to bed for several months. The study found that the students lost about 10 per cent of their muscle bulk and strength in the first week of bed rest, and even more over subsequent weeks.

If you stay in, sitting down or lying in bed, you can begin to feel weaker, and stiffen up. This is especially true when one lies down or sits in a chair for many hours non-stop.

But the good news is that a slow, steady increase in activity can help improve your physical flexibility. And any pain caused by resting too much will slowly reduce. This is why physiotherapists and doctors advise people to try to maintain activity levels as much as possible. This is especially important if you have had to rest to begin with, for example, after having a caesarean. You need to slowly rebuild activities at a sensible pace as your scar heals.

Example: Sally's reduced activities

Sally has had postnatal depression for the past nine months. She has felt increasingly tired and worn out. She is sleeping poorly and has found everything a struggle. Because of how she feels she has started to do less and less. She stays in most of the time with her son Jack, and now only goes out to go to the supermarket. She has stopped meeting most of her friends.

Whenever someone from her antenatal group phones up to say they are having a get-together she says she has something on that day and can't make it. She then feels guilty afterwards for lying. During the day she does what she has to, looks after Jack and then just sits watching TV. She looks around the house at all the things that need to be done – the washing, cooking and cleaning – and feels overwhelmed. Where can she even start? She sits crying just thinking about it, but also gets angry whenever her partner John suggests they book a cleaner to help her. She thinks 'I should be able to do this myself'. Overall she feels she is failing.

Now think about your own life.

Do you have a similar pattern of reduced activity? Write what you haven't been doing below.

Based on your reply above, overall, have you stopped doing things you used to enjoy as a result of how you feel?

Yes ☐   No ☐   Sometimes ☐

Q Has the reduced activity:

- Removed things from your life that previously gave you a sense of pleasure/achievement?

Yes ☐   No ☐   Sometimes ☐

- Or worsened how you feel physically?

Yes ☐   No ☐   Sometimes ☐

Q Overall, has this worsened how you feel?

Yes ☐   No ☐   Sometimes ☐

If you have answered 'Yes' or 'Sometimes' to all the questions above, then reduced activity is causing a problem for you. This workbook will help you find out how to overcome reduced activity.

First steps to boosting how you feel

The plan first is to discover:

- The things you've done in the past that you know make you feel good.
- The things you are doing that give you a boost.

So you need to keep a **record** of what you are currently doing. An *activity diary* can help you do this. After that you should rate **each** activity you do every day (see pages 188–189).

What activities should you record?

Use the activity diary at the end of the workbook to record **everything** that you do over the next few days. For example:

- Getting dressed.
- Getting your baby up.
- Doing some housework.
- Going out shopping.

- Washing your baby.

- Dressing your baby.

- Feeding your baby.

- Playing with your baby.

- Listening to the radio.

- Having a shower.

- Having breakfast yourself.

- Chatting to your partner.

- Washing your hair.

- Doing the washing up etc.

Also include times when you are sitting and watching TV, having a bath or resting etc. In other words try to record **everything** – you are probably doing far more than you thought.

Rating your activities

Remember to **be fair on yourself** when judging how much of a sense of achievement an activity gives you. If you are struggling at the moment, it's a big achievement if you and your baby get up, get washed and get dressed. Don't think 'Well I should be able to do that anyway'. Even when someone is struggling to maintain the activities they did before, it's likely that some life activities will continue to provide a sense of pleasure, achievement or closeness to others.

Using the graph overleaf, rate your activities as follows:

1. The **pleasure or fun** you have while doing the activity (0–10 scale).

2. How much of an **achievement** it was (0–10 scale). In other words were you able to look back with satisfaction and think that it was a job well done?

3. How **close** you felt to people or your baby, again rated on a 0–10 scale.

No pleasure or fun	Felt OK	Complete pleasure or fun
No achievement	Felt OK	Complete achievement
No sense of closeness	Felt OK	Complete sense of closeness

```
L___|___|___|___|___|___|___|___|___|___J
0    1    2    3    4    5    6    7    8    9    10
```

Example: Sally rates her activities

Sally goes out for a walk with the pram and gives this a score of 5/10 for pleasure. She also rates this activity as 7/10 for achievement (she didn't want to go, and it felt difficult, but she managed it). She also rates herself as 8/10 for closeness as she felt closer to Jack as she pulled faces and smiled as they walked.

For an example of a completed diary, see Sally's activity diary on the next page. This shows that even though she is doing less than she used to she is still doing lots of things. Importantly, several of these activities can help her feel better.

Example: Sally's activity diary

Date and time	Activity (include everything you do)	How long did you do it for?	Pleasure felt 0 = no pleasure 10 = maximum pleasure	How much of an achievement was it given how you feel? 0 = no sense of achievement 10 = maximum sense of achievement	How much of a sense of closeness did you feel? 0 = no sense of closeness 10 = maximum sense of closeness
6–7 am	In bed, asleep	7 hours!	1	1	1
7–8 am	Jack started crying. Brought him into my bed and fed him	30 minutes	3	3	6
8–9 am	Got up and had a shower, cleaned my teeth. Got Jack changed	40 minutes	3	6	6
9–10 am	Made a coffee and had some toast	15 minutes	5	5	5
10–11 am	Watched television	90 minutes	4	2	2
11–12 pm	Watched television	50 minutes	5	2	2
12–1 pm	Did the ironing	45 minutes	6	8	8

0	1	2	3	4	5	6	7	8	9	10

No pleasure or fun — Felt OK — Complete pleasure or fun
No achievement — Felt OK — Complete achievement
No sense of closeness — Felt OK — Complete sense of closeness

Task

Now start keeping an activity diary yourself and continue for the next few days. Use the blank diary at the back of this workbook to tear out or copy. Don't forget to include what you're doing at the moment – reading the workbook!

Use the diary to discover **patterns** in what you do and don't do. Later, you will also use the diary to help you to work out a first target to change.

Key point

The aim of keeping a diary is to help you to find out which activities or situations make you feel better. This allows you to plan to do more similar things in your life.

How the activity diary can help you move forwards

The all-or-nothing approach

Sometimes it can be tempting to introduce changes into your life too quickly. If you find that you've got into a habit of doing very little – and then suddenly throw yourself into doing too much – things can backfire. **Overdoing things can sometimes be just as unhelpful as under-doing.** This is called the **all-or-nothing** response (see the solid line in the figure below). The person throws themselves into things on days when they feel better. The problem is that they then crash back. The result is that on average they do less and less – as shown by the dotted line.

The all-or-nothing cycle – overdoing things in ways that backfire.

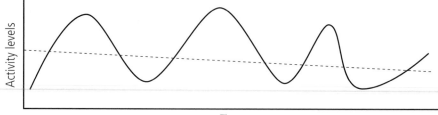

Now think about your own self – if you feel good one day, do you then tend to try to do too many things, leaving you feeling exhausted for the next few days? This can also happen when you have a good week and feel almost back to your usual self. This **all-or-nothing** cycle usually happens not only when you're feeling your worst but also when you are recovering. It can be very frustrating and makes it hard to plan your life.

For example, if you are ironing the clothes, taking a paced approach would include a break halfway through and maybe finishing later that day. In contrast, taking an 'all-or-nothing' approach would mean that the person throws themselves into doing it all at once – exhausting themselves in the process as illustrated below.

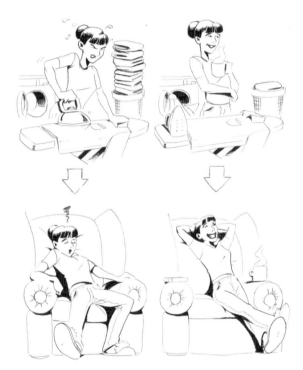

The paced approach

Once you have an idea of your current activity level you can build on this to pace yourself and increase your activity levels. You use the same activity diary and complete it in advance with a plan of what you will do.

For some people this may mean that at first you might actually **reduce** what you are currently doing. This can feel strange because, for example, like Sally, on some days you may be able to do all of the washing and most of the ironing. Other days you may find it really hard to get up and do any laundry at all. A better situation would therefore be to do some every day. So by using a 'pacing' approach to change your behaviour you can break the 'all-or-nothing' cycle.

Overcoming reduced activity

Setting targets can help you make the changes needed to get better in a planned way. To do this you will need to decide:

- **Short-term** targets – these are changes you can make today, tomorrow and the next week.
- **Medium-term** targets – these are the changes to be put in place over the next few weeks.
- **Long-term** targets – this is where you want to be in six months or a year.

The seven-step plan

The best way to change things is to slowly increase **specific** activities to boost your confidence and feelings of pleasure and achievement.

Step 1: Identify and clearly define the problem

By now, you will already have an idea of the different activities you are doing – and not doing – from your activity diary.

The following table lists the activities that are commonly affected when you have low mood or depression. You will probably have noticed changes in at least some of these activities.

Checklist: Identifying your patterns of reduced activity

As a result of how you feel, are you:	Tick here if you have noticed this – even if just sometimes
Stopping or reducing doing hobbies/interests such as reading or other things you previously enjoyed or did to relax?	☐
Going out or meeting friends less than usual?	☐
Eating poorly (for example eating less or tending to eat more 'junk' food, or food that takes little preparation)?	☐
Noticing physical consequences of reduced activity – such as worsened stiffness/pain, restricted joint movement or slowly worsening weakness of under-used muscles?	☐
Brooding over things and therefore no longer living life to the full?	☐
Failing to keep up with housework (for example are you 'letting things go' around the house)?	☐
Not always answering the phone or the door when people visit?	☐
Leaving letters/bills unopened or not replying to them because of a lack of energy or interest in actively dealing with them?	☐
Paying less attention to your self-care or personal hygiene (for example washing less, less bothered about your appearance, leaving clothes on for longer, not shaving, or not combing your hair)?	☐
Less interested in sex (for example pushing your partner away physically because of a lack of enjoyment/energy for sex)?	☐
Staying inactive or lying in bed so that you are far less physically active than before?	☐
If you have a religious faith: have you reduced or stopped reading your Holy book, praying or going to meetings?	☐

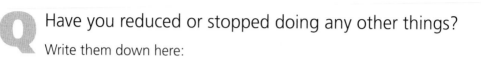 Have you reduced or stopped doing any other things?

Write them down here:

Look back at your list and your diary and from these choose a **single** target to change first. This is particularly important if you have ticked several boxes in the checklist. It isn't possible to overcome all these areas at once.

Instead you need to decide on **one** area to concentrate on.

Example: Sally's activities

Look back at Sally's example on page 165. Sally is doing far less than before. From her diary she has noticed several things that gave her more feelings of pleasure, achievement or closeness.

Sally decides that she wants to focus on keeping up with the housework. She chooses this because she knows it upsets her. She even lies awake at night worrying about how everything is so out of hand. This then is her first target.

Choosing a first target

Write down the one problem area you want to work on here:

(Remember that this should be a problem of reduced activity that is worsening how you feel.)

Be a detective

The next thing is to do some research on what stops you doing things. First, record in detail every time you put off doing something over several days. Try to work out what makes things hard:

- The time of day.

- Whether you have slept well the night before.

- Who you were with and how they responded.

- How you felt emotionally.

- What went through your mind.

- How you felt emotionally and physically at the time.

… and anything else that seems to help explain your reaction.

Now use your investigations to decide whether you need to break your target into smaller steps. If you do, write down your first target again:

Check point: Is this a realistic target for change?

Remember that you should have written a small, focused problem that you can work on. You need to remember that any change you make not only needs to push you but also needs to be realistic and achievable.

Now check if it's a realistic target by answering the following **Questions for effective change**.

Q Is your target:

- Clear and realistic and something you can tackle over the next week or two?

Yes ☐   No ☐

- Not so scary that you can't face doing it?

Yes ☐   No ☐

- Still big enough to move you forwards?

Yes ☐   No ☐

Example: Sally breaks her target into smaller steps

Sally has decided to focus on doing the housework. This is quite a general problem – as there are so many different possible bits of the housework she could do (ironing, vacuuming, dusting, cleaning out cupboards, etc). In fact there is so much that she looks at the target and feels overwhelmed. She knows that her spare time is quite limited because Jack needs feeding and attention a lot of the time. Whatever she does needs to be fitted into times when Jack is asleep or sitting quietly in his rocker.

Sally goes through the questions for effective change and decides her target isn't clear and realistic enough. So she breaks it down into smaller tasks. She decides to start by focusing on the ironing.

Q Do you need to break your target down into a number of smaller, more achievable targets?

Yes ☐   No ☐

If you answered 'Yes', go straight to Step 2. If you answered 'No', then keep reading about how to choose a realistic first target.

Go back to thinking about your problem. What smaller steps could help you move forwards? If you need to, rewrite your first target again.

My clear first step is:

Step 2: Think up as many solutions as possible to achieve your first goal

Try to come up with as many ideas as possible. Completely whacky ideas should be included as well even if you would never choose them in practice. Try to **think broadly**. The following questions will help you come up with ideas:

 What advice would you give a friend who was trying to tackle the same problem?

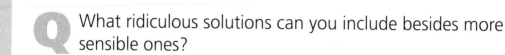 What ridiculous solutions can you include besides more sensible ones?

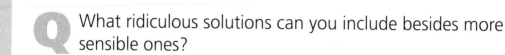 What helpful suggestions would others make?

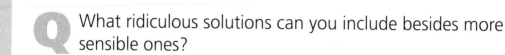 How could you look at the solutions facing you differently? What would you have said before you felt like this, or what might you say about the situation say in five years' time?

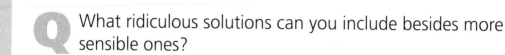 What approaches have you tried in the past in similar circumstances?

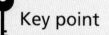
Key point

If you feel stuck, sometimes doing this task with someone you trust can help.

Example: Sally's ideas

I could:

- Employ a full-time helper, who could do the ironing – and everything else as well!
- Iron everything in one fell swoop.
- Break it down into chunks – and do five or six things when I can.
- Use an ironing service.
- Try to iron a bit more with Jack there in his musical rocker.

Now it's your turn. Write down as many possible options (including ridiculous ideas at first) to help you tackle your problem:

Step 3: Look at the pros and cons of each possible solution

Example: Sally's list of pros and cons

Idea	Pros (advantages)	Cons (disadvantages)
Employ a full time helper who could do the ironing – and everything else as well!	They could do it all – including all the other things	Well, we've no money for a start. And it would be embarrassing
Iron everything in one fell swoop	It would get it all out of the way – IF I could do it	There's too much – at least 40–50 items. I haven't got long before something happens. Jack's always needing something
Break it down into chunks – and do five or six things when I can	That's a great idea. I often have time when I could do five or six things. That's very realistic. It would all add up if I could do that each day	It would be a pain putting the ironing board up and down
Use an ironing service	I don't like paying other people for things I can do myself	They are expensive, and there's all the hassle of getting the items there. They can pick things up but this costs extra. We don't really have the money. I'd feel embarrassed
Try to iron a bit more with Jack there in his musical rocker	That's another great idea. He loves sitting and bouncing in his rocker, and the music and lights keep him interested. I could smile and make noises to distract him if he gets upset – and keep ironing	There's not many downsides. I'd get the ironing done and it doesn't depend on Jack being asleep

Write your own list of ideas into the following table with pros and cons of each suggestion.

My suggestions from Step 2	Pros (advantages)	Cons (disadvantages)

Step 4: Now choose one of the solutions

Your chosen solution should be an option that will make a sensible first step in tackling your problem. It should be realistic and likely to succeed. The decision needs to be based on all your answers to Step 3.

In making your decision, bear in mind that the best way of tackling reduced activity is to plan **steady, slow changes**.

Key point

The solution you are looking for is something that gets you moving in the right direction. This should be small enough to be possible, but big enough to move you forwards.

Example: Sally's chosen solution

Sally decides to try to iron a bit more when Jack is in his musical rocker.

Now look at your responses in Step 3 and then choose a solution.

Write down your preferred solution here:

Now see if you can answer 'Yes' to the three **Questions for effective change** below:

Q Will it be *useful* for changing how you are?

Yes ☐   No ☐

Q Is it a *clear* **task** so that you will know when you have done it?

Yes ☐   No ☐

Q Is it something that is realistic, practical and achievable?

Yes ☐   No ☐

Step 5: Plan the steps needed to carry out your chosen solution

You need to have a clear plan that lays out exactly **what** you are going to do and **when** you are going to do it. **Write down** the steps needed to carry out your plan. This will help you to think what to do and also to predict possible problems that might arise. Remember that an important part of the planning process is also to predict what would block the plan. That way you can think about how you will respond if there were problems to keep your plan on track.

Example: Sally's plan

Sally decides that she will carry out her plan in the afternoon after Jack wakes up and has had a feed. She knows Jack tends to be most settled then. She plans to bring the ironing board into the lounge as well as the ironing. There's a power plug there and an extension wire to plug the iron in. She also plans to bring only five items through to iron. That way Sally knows she won't feel upset by what's not done. She decides she will iron as long as she can – but not for more than 20 items. That way she can avoid overly throwing herself into things. She will pop Jack safely in his musical rocker and switch it on.

Sally also thinks about what might block the plan. If Jack is out of sorts and screams she will need to break off and give him a cuddle, settle him and then try again. If someone comes to the door she will need to break off, and if they stay then plan to do it the next day. Finally, Sally is aware that sometimes she feels so tired she doesn't fancy doing things. She decides therefore to tell John that morning that she is going to do some of the ironing. She has learned that telling someone else she is going to do something can help keep her motivated to do it.

Now, write down your plan here:

Q What will you do if something happens to block your plan?

Write down what you could do to unblock your plan:

Now check your plan against the rest of the **Questions for effective change**.

Q Is your plan one that:

- Makes clear what you are going to do and when you are going to do it?

  Yes ☐   No ☐

- Won't be easily blocked or prevented by practical problems?

  Yes ☐   No ☐

- Will help you to learn useful things even if it doesn't work out perfectly?

  Yes ☐   No ☐

Step 6: Carry out your plan

Now carry out your plan during the next week.

Pay attention to your thoughts about what will happen before, during and after you have completed your plan.

Write any thoughts/fears you noticed here:

Try to do your plan anyway. Good luck!

Step 7: Review the outcome

Example: Did Sally's plan work?

Sally gets everything set up. She manages two shirts then Jack starts shouting. Sally stops ironing and gives him a cuddle. Jack gives a large burp and then settles. Sally pops Jack back in the rocker and starts ironing again.

She manages to quickly finish the first five items and then goes for another five. She gets through 14 items in total and thinks 'This is great'. She finally manages to finish ironing 18 items before Jack starts complaining and she has to stop. Sally is pleased she had set things up so she could feel good every five items rather than being annoyed she didn't manage 'the full 20'. She also was pleased because she felt close to Jack – and was able to pull faces and giggle at him as she ironed.

Now write down your review:

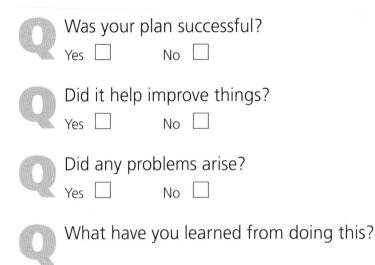

Was your plan successful?

Yes ☐   No ☐

Did it help improve things?

Yes ☐   No ☐

Did any problems arise?

Yes ☐   No ☐

What have you learned from doing this?

Write down any helpful lessons or information you have learned from what happened. If things didn't go quite as you hoped, try to learn from what happened.

How could you make things different during your next attempt to tackle the problem?

Were you too ambitious or unrealistic in choosing the target you did?

Planning the next steps

Now that you have reviewed how your first planned activity went, the next step is to plan another activity to build on this. You need to think again about your **short**, **medium** and **longer-term** targets. Did your plan help you completely tackle the area of reduced activity you were working on? You may need to plan out other solutions to tackle different aspects of your problem. The key is to build one step upon another.

Each step should again be realistic, practical and achievable. Without a step-by-step approach you may find that although you take some steps forward, these are all in different directions and you lose your focus and motivation. Use what you have just learned to build on what you did.

Example: Sally's short, medium and longer-term targets

Short-term – what might Sally do over the next week or so? This is the next step she needs to plan.

Sally's target: I want to keep working on the ironing until I am up to date with it.

Medium term – what might you aim towards doing over the next few weeks – the next few steps?

Sally's target: I want to keep up to date with the ironing, but also move on to tidying rooms one at a time. For the larger rooms I'm going to break this down into smaller tasks. I'll tidy them a bit, then a bit more the next day. Then build in the vacuuming. I'll plan just two times a week at this – I can't do everything – I've got a young baby.

Longer-term: where do you want to be in a few months or so?

Sally's target: I want to get a balance. I need to accept that I can't keep things as clean and neat as I used to before Jack was born. If John wants things any tidier he needs to do it himself! I know I can keep up with two to three short ironing sessions a week, and one to two short cleaning sessions. That's something nearly every day. I'll keep planning to do this using my activity diary. If something comes up and I can't do it on a particular day, I won't beat myself up but just do it the next day.

Now it's your turn. In creating your plan:

Do:

- Plan to alter **only** one or two things over the next week.

- Plan to alter things slowly in a step-by-step way.

- Use the **Questions for effective change** to check that the next step is always well planned.

- Write down your plan in detail so that you know exactly what you are going to do this week.

Don't:

- Try to start to alter too many things all at once.

- Choose something that is too hard a target to start with.

- Be very negative and think 'It's a waste of time'. Try to experiment to find out if this negative thinking is actually true.

Write your own short, medium and long-term plans here:

- **Short-term** – what might you do over the next week or so? This is the next step you need to plan.

- **Medium-term** – what might you aim towards doing over the next few weeks – the next few steps?

- **Longer-term** – where do you want to be in a few months or so?

Remember to plan slow, steady changes. This will help you to rebuild your confidence, as you tackle your avoidance. You'll also probably realise that facing fears is one of the best ways of tackling your worries as well.

Summary

In this workbook you have:

- Learnt how low mood and stress causes you to do less.
- Found out how reduced activity affects you.
- Recorded your current activity levels and discovered what gives you a boost.
- Planned ways to make slow, steady changes to your life to boost how you feel.
- Planned some next steps to build on these changes.

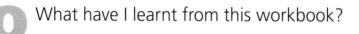 What have I learnt from this workbook?

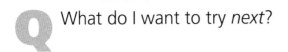

What do I want to try *next*?

Putting what you have learned into practice

📌 Task

Plan some action plans over the next few weeks to tackle your reduced activity. If you have problems just try to change things using slow, steady steps.

Good luck!

Acknowledgements

I wish to thank all those who have commented upon this workbook, especially Dr Nicky Dummett and Catriona Kent.

My notes

Activity Diary/Planner (1 of 2)

Date and time	Activity (include everything you do)	How long did you do it for?	Pleasure felt 0 = no pleasure 10 = maximum pleasure	How much of an achievement was it given how you feel? 0 = no sense of achievement 10 = maximum sense of achievement	Sense of closeness to others 0 = no sense of closeness 10 = maximum sense of closeness
6–7 am					
7–8 am					
8–9 am					
9–10 am					
10–11 am					
11–12 pm					
12–1 pm					
1–2 pm					
2–3 pm					
3–4 pm					

Activity Diary/Planner (2 of 2)

Date and time	Activity (include everything you do)	How long did you do it for?	Pleasure felt 0 = no pleasure 10 = maximum pleasure	How much of an achievement was it given how you feel? 0 = no sense of achievement 10 = maximum sense of achievement	Sense of closeness to others 0 = no sense of closeness 10 = maximum sense of closeness
4–5 pm					
5–6 pm					
6–7 pm					
7–8 pm					
8–9 pm					
9–10 pm					
10–11 pm					
11–12 am					
Later					

Overcoming Postnatal Depression

A Five Areas Approach

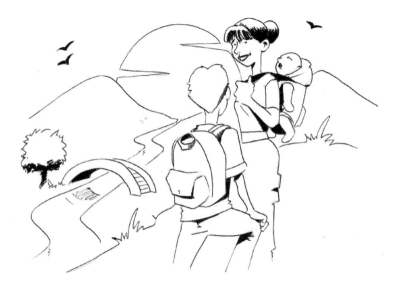

Using exercise to boost how you feel

www.livinglifetothefull.com
www.fiveareas.com

Dr Chris Williams, Dr Roch Cantwell and Karen Robertson

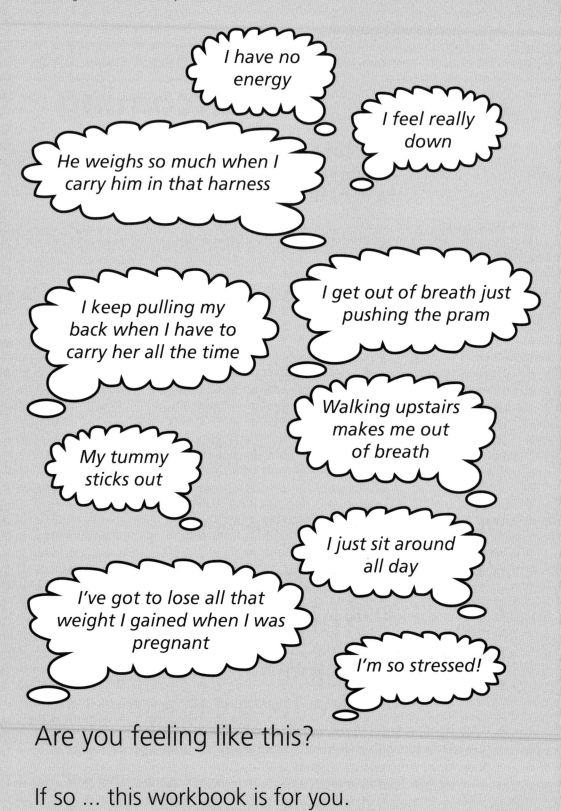

Are you feeling like this?

If so ... this workbook is for you.

Why bother with exercise?

Your emotions, thinking, behaviour, relationships, life situation and your body all affect each other. They are all connected. Therefore increasing **your physical activity levels can boost how you feel** mentally as well as physically. But people often forget to exercise when they feel unwell or it seems too hard.

Think about a time when you had a bad cold. Besides a runny nose and a sore throat – did you feel subdued, fed-up and down emotionally as well?

Now think back to a time when you exercised – such as riding a bike, running or swimming. Some people find that they often get a **mental 'high'** after exercise. However, having a baby can affect your ability to maintain your previous activity levels. You just may not have the time (or the money) to do things such as going to a gym.

In this workbook you will:

- See how exercise can boost your mood.

- Learn how to use exercise to reduce your tension and anxiety.

- Discover how exercise can help you feel fitter, more active and better about yourself.

Why exercise may be good for you

People often forget to exercise when they feel unwell or it seems too hard. So exercise can be 'prescribed' by doctors as part of treatment for depression.

- Exercise can be fun if you choose something that you have previously liked doing.

- It gives **you** control to plan things at your own pace.

- It can help you structure and plan your day – rather than just staying in and being inactive.

- It can boost your social life. Doing things with others such as a step class, going for a run with your friends, playing football or going for a swim can help you meet others with a shared interest.

- Even with a baby you can think of exercise. Check out whether there are any aqua-aerobics or mother/baby exercise and massage classes in your area.

- Walking with the pram (and another mum) is also good exercise.

It really is a win-win situation.

Are there any downsides of exercise?

- If you have had a caesarean section, you may not be able to do certain exercises for a time. Ask your doctor or health visitor for advice about what you can or can't do over the first month or two after having your baby.

- You may have aching muscles to begin with!

- There can be a cost for some activities (for example, for using a gym or a swimming pool).

- It's also best not to take your baby swimming until after their first immunisation injections.

How planned exercise can help you feel better

Experiment

You'll need less than 15 minutes to do this experiment. The aim is to test if even a small amount of exercise affects how you feel overall.

Before you start think of a physical activity that you can do. This should be something:

- That is realistic, bearing in mind how you are physically at the moment.

- That can be done in just 5–10 minutes to start with.

- You know is within your capabilities and doesn't push you.

Please choose something just now that doesn't involve vigorous exercise.

Here's an example. Walk up and down a flight of stairs three to four times. Take a rest if you get out of breath.

Key point

This isn't asking you to do a workout. You don't need to get changed, work up a sweat or even do warm-up exercises!

Other things you could try are stretching your body, jogging slowly on the spot or walking round the block with the pram at a reasonable pace. Remember not to overdo it. Aim to do something that gets your heart rate up and gets you moving **without being excessive**. Remember, any benefits can be boosted even more by planning to do activities that are fun or sociable. If you think you're physically unwell you can always check this with your doctor first.

Doing your planned exercise

So you've chosen what to do. **Before you start** put a cross on the two lines below to show how you feel right now.

How I feel now

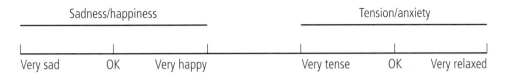

Now do your 5–10 minutes' exercise. Remember you can stop for a rest if you feel this is too long for you.

Your review

Immediately afterwards please rate your mood again.

How I feel after my exercise

After your exercise:

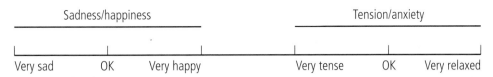

Next: stop, think and reflect

Have a look at your scores before and after.

Task

Q Did you notice any changes? Write down any changes you noticed in your thoughts/mental energy/how positive you feel/your ability to think clearly:

Q How did you feel during the task? Write down how you felt emotionally (tension, anger, stress, sadness, happiness, enthusiasm):

Q How did you feel physically? Write down how you felt physically (relaxed/tense, jittery, tired, achy, ready for more):

Write down any other changes you noticed:

Q Overall, do you think you might benefit from planning some exercise into your life as part of your own 'mental fitness' package.

Yes ☐   No ☐   Yes, but ... ☐

Yes, but ...

There are often lots of things in life that we know are good for us, but we don't do them. Remember, that's just as true in other people's lives as it may be in your own.

Tackling the simple blocks

Often the biggest problems are simple ones:

• Perhaps you just aren't in the habit of doing exercise.

• Or maybe you want to get into the habit of doing exercise but it proves hard. For example it's easy for us to talk ourselves out of it. This is a common problem.

Many people see exercise as too hard or boring, too expensive, taking too much time – or all of these!

Q **What thoughts block you from doing exercise?**

Write them down here:

But planning to do exercise doesn't mean you have to make a big change to your lifestyle. Even **small changes** can make a positive difference. Now find a way to make this easier for yourself, for example, fitting it into what you already do each day.

Key point

Exercise and injury: Remember it's important to **warm-up to avoid muscle pulls, aches and strains**. Using good techniques and the right equipment, clothing and shoes is also important.

Making a clear plan that works for you

People are often amazed at how empowering, energising and good it can feel when they get into the habit of exercising as part of their regular daily routine.

- Choose something that gets you going physically.

- Build up the amount of exercise slowly in a gradual and planned way.

- Don't throw yourself into things too quickly (or start too slowly): **pacing is the key**.

- Many people find that doing exercise towards the start of the day helps them to 'get going'. Try to avoid exercising just before going to bed as this can unhelpfully affect your sleep.

- Look to do this with help. Plan to exercise with a friend.

- Remember that walking with your baby, talking to them about what you see as you walk and doing this with a friend is a good example of cheap and effective exercise.

- If you've signed up to the **www.livinglifetothefull.com** course you'll get short **email reminders** to help keep you on track. This course is free and you can cancel at any time. Please note the course doesn't offer advice on an individual basis.

Planning when and how to exercise

Exercising on a regular basis – even if it is just a short time to begin with – is important. It is often helpful to actively plan this into your day and diary rather than just 'trying to fit it in some time'. You may find the following **planning task** helpful in making this regular commitment.

My plan to use exercise to help me feel better

Q **What** am I going to do?

(Remember to choose something that is possible, realistic and achievable. Preferably choose something that is fun. Think about planning some exercise that has a social aspect at least once a week, for example pushing the pram with a friend (and your baby!), a step or yoga class or going for a run or walk with friends. Remember exercise doesn't need to cost lots of money. You can get exercise videos and DVDs for a small weekly charge from your local library. Or you could walk to your local shop each time instead of taking the bus or being driven.)

Q **When** am I going to plan to do some exercise?

(Think about whether doing some exercise every day is practical for you. If it is, what time of day would be best for you? If you can't manage it every day then how about just once or twice a week? You can always build upon this at a later stage.)

Q **How much** exercise will I do?

(Be realistic – think about your current level of fitness, health and motivation. If you have doubts about your health, please discuss this with your doctor.)

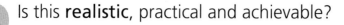

Is this **realistic**, practical and achievable?

(You know your own life and its various demands and commitments.)

What problems could prevent me doing this, and how can I overcome them?

(For example your baby's routine, work or family deadlines such as meeting other children from school, money, or having the kit you need.)

Keeping on track

Once you have created your exercise plan it is **important to keep on track**. This means setting yourself goals and reviewing your progress. In this way you can make changes if things aren't going well.

My plan for the next few weeks

(Think about short-term, medium-term and long-term changes.)

What are you going to do?

How will you try to make sure that you carry out your plan?

 When are you going to do it?

 What can stop this happening?

(What problems might there be, and how can you overcome them? What might sabotage your plan?)

Date of my next review (review your plan monthly, set aside a time to do this. Put it into your schedule or diary):

Summary

In this workbook you have learned:

- How exercise can boost how you feel.
- The benefits and 'side effects' of exercise.
- Ways of planning exercise into your life in a paced way.

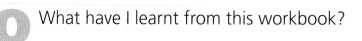 What have I learnt from this workbook?

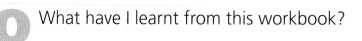 What do I want to try *next*?

Putting things into practice

Read this module again and then plan your own exercise. Try to stick to your plan.

Other sources of support

- Your GP may be able to refer you to an exercise class you can attend free of charge.

- Look out for classes for you and your baby at your local swimming pool or gym. Some pools and gyms also have crèches.

- Think about tennis, badminton or walking classes.

- Find out more: the Mental Health Foundation provides useful information on its website about exercise and mood (see **www.mentalhealth.org.uk**).

- Do it with a friend! Plan to do exercise with a friend or colleague.

 Do the online module about healthy living at **www.livinglifetothefull.com**.

My notes

Overcoming Postnatal Depression
A Five Areas Approach

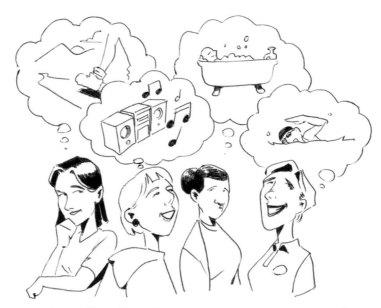

Helpful things you do

www.livinglifetothefull.com
www.fiveareas.com

Dr Chris Williams, Dr Roch Cantwell and
Karen Robertson

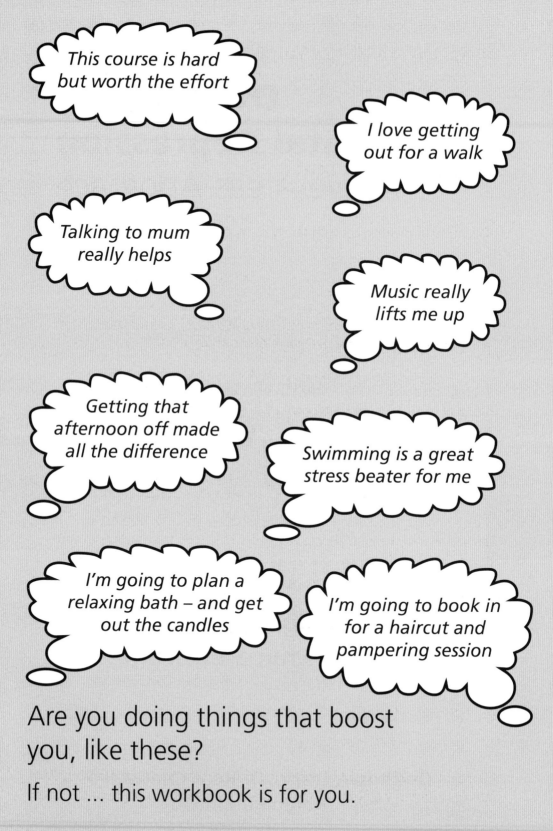

Are you doing things that boost you, like these?

If not ... this workbook is for you.

> # In this workbook you will:
>
> - Learn about helpful things you can do that can give you a boost.
>
> - Plan some ways to make sure that you do these things, even when you are busy.

What are helpful activities?

Helpful activities include:

- Talking to or meeting up with family or friends.

- Doing things that give you a boost, for example getting outside, walking in the park, reading a book or going swimming – all the things that often fall by the wayside when you first have a baby.

- Pampering yourself, such as having a special bath with music and candles, or a nice meal, a haircut or something else you enjoy. It doesn't have to be costly.

- Finding out about how to tackle low mood in postnatal depression. For example, reading books like this one, or reading information leaflets and factsheets you can get from charities and other organisations that support women with postnatal depression. A list of these is given at the end of the *Understanding why you feel as you do* workbook.

- Seeing your GP to find out what support is available for you locally, for example, whether you should see an expert mental health worker.

- Keeping going – activity helps overcome low mood. Get outside, try to meet people and say hello to people you know as you go for a walk with your baby. All these things will give you a boost and help you stay confident.

📌 Task

Write down any *helpful* things you have done here in the past two weeks.

You may not have thought of this, but it makes sense to plan these things into your week. In this way you will give yourself little boosts throughout the week.

What are you doing that helps give you a boost?

Are you:	Tick here if you have noticed this – even if just sometimes
Being good to yourself?	☐
For example, eating regularly and healthily; taking time to enjoy the food	
Doing things for fun/pleasure?	☐
For example, your hobbies, listening to music, having a nice bath – with the whole candles thing!	
Seeking support from others whom you trust?	☐
For example, seeking out other helpful sources of support, like going to a self-help group meeting (your GP can tell you about these groups)	
Keeping in touch with others even if you don't feel like it?	☐
Pick a level of contact you can cope with, for example by telephone, email or meeting up	
Playing with your baby, and spending time together having cuddles?	☐
Stopping, thinking and reflecting on things rather than jumping to conclusions?	☐
For example, letting upsetting thoughts 'just be' rather than mulling over them	
Finding out more about postnatal depression by reading information leaflets, self-help books etc., that is putting what you have learned into practice?	☐
Doing too much or too little?	☐
Pace yourself – so you don't run out of energy or sit doing very little	

Are you:	Tick here if you have noticed this – even if just sometimes
Planning time for yourself, or you and your partner together without the baby?	☐
For example, you can plan to leave your baby with a friend, relative or crèche while you spend time for yourself. For example talking/doing adult things like going out for a meal	
Keeping as active as you can?	☐
For example, doing exercise/going for walks/swimming/pottering round the garden/going to a gym. After your baby is three months old, you can take them to the swimming pool. Think of baby swimming sessions/baby aqua-aerobics	
Note: If you had a caesarean or your back or front hip joints are painful after the birth, you need to take it easy for a few weeks. But once your doctor or GP says it's okay, try to keep reasonably active. If you rest too much you will find you feel stiffer and more easily tired. Try walking with as relaxed and normal a posture as possible	
Using your sense of humour to cope?	☐
For example, let's face it – babies create a lot of sick and poo and you need that sense of humour	
Giving yourself a break?	☐
Remember: no-one is the perfect mother or father!	
Taking any prescribed medication regularly and as prescribed?	☐
Remember that the medication is there to help.	

Overcoming Postnatal Depression: A Five Areas Approach

Are you:	Tick here if you have noticed this – even if just sometimes
Trying using things such as relaxation tapes, slow breathing, etc. to deal with tension (see **www.livinglifetothefull.com** and MP3 downloads at **www.fiveareas.com**)	☐
For example, if you have a partner, try swapping relaxing massages that don't necessarily lead to sex	
Being honest with trusted others (especially your GP) about how you really are?	☐
If you are struggling you need to say so, otherwise people will not know you need help.	

List any other helpful behaviours you do here:

Now think about your answers:

Q **Are you doing any helpful things that boost how you feel?**

Yes ☐   No ☐   Sometimes ☐

(If you answered 'No', you'll have an opportunity to plan some helpful activity later in the workbook.)

Q **Do the helpful things you do help in the short and longer term?**

Yes ☐   No ☐   Sometimes ☐

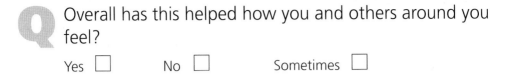 Overall has this helped how you and others around you feel?

Yes ☐   No ☐   Sometimes ☐

If you have answered 'Yes' or 'Sometimes' to these questions, you are responding to people and events around you in some helpful ways. Well done! Building these helpful responses into your life is an important way of feeling better.

When helpful things can become unhelpful

Sometimes you think that an activity is helpful, but in fact it's part of the problem. For example:

● Drinking a lot.

● Avoiding people and events around you.

● Seeking reassurance.

Key point

Many helpful things you do can become unhelpful for you or for others if you rely on them too much or do them all the time.

Some things that may seem helpful but can backfire if you do them too much

Drinking

Having a small glass of alcohol might be quite normal when you are socialising. But drinking too much during pregnancy, or afterwards, can backfire for:

● You: you can get headaches, feel ill, put on weight, make unwise decisions, or your depression can worsen.

● Your baby: if you have too much alcohol when you are pregnant it can damage your growing baby. But alcohol also gets into breast milk so can harm the baby after birth. Besides this, mothers who drink too much could end up neglecting their baby or harming them.

● Others around you, for example your partner, friends or family members: if alcohol becomes a problem these are the people on the receiving end who will have to pick up the pieces.

The *Alcohol, drugs and your baby* workbook can help if alcohol or drugs are an issue for you.

Seeking reassurance

Sharing problems and talking things through with people you trust can really help. But if you look to others for support all the time, and contact them again and again for every little thing you do, they may get frustrated. This can end up undermining your confidence. So what you need is a balanced, supportive relationship.

Seeking (or receiving) too much help from others

Sometimes people may offer 'helpful advice' all the time and want to do **everything** for you. There can be many reasons for this such as being concerned about you, or your friendship and love. Or sometimes it may be because the other person feels anxious or even guilty about your low mood.

Whatever the cause, you may feel suffocated and frustrated. Or you may feel that you are being treated like a child. This can sap your confidence, or annoy you and lead to arguments. And little irritations can quickly build up. The workbook *Information for family and friends – how can you offer the best support?* has some helpful suggestions for you and any of your family and friends to help deal with such issues.

You can find out more about how to overcome these three unhelpful behaviours and more in the workbook *Unhelpful things you do*.

Now let's move on to possible ways in which you can build helpful behaviours into your life.

Building helpful responses

Some activities may seem quite easy to do right away. Others may need some formal planning using the seven-step plan below.

Step 1: Choose one helpful activity you plan to do

Go back to the checklist on pages 208–210. Choose an activity that you would like to do. You can choose any, but it's often helpful to choose things you know from previous experience can help.

Write down your chosen helpful activity here:

Example: Julia's helpful activity

Julia has postnatal depression. She knows that meeting up with others gives her a boost. She decides she will plan some time with her friends.

Step 2: Think up as many ways as possible to do your planned activity

Here's where you need to come up with as many ideas as possible. Try to **think broadly**. For a start, think of some whacky ideas as well, even if you would never choose to do them.

The following questions can help you with possible ideas:

- What advice would you give a friend who was trying to make the same changes? Sometimes we can more easily think of solutions for others than for ourselves.

- What *ridiculous* solutions can you include as well as more sensible ones?

- What helpful ideas would others (for example family, friends or colleagues) suggest?

- What have you tried in the past that was helpful?

Key point

If you feel stuck, sometimes doing this task with someone you trust can be helpful.

> ## 🔍 Example: Julia's helpful ideas
>
> - First a crazy idea – I could fly everyone out to a desert island!
> - I could invite some friends for lunch.
> - I could invite one or two friends for a walk in the park.
> - I could do something with others and leave Ben with someone like mum.
> - I could have a children's party and invite all the adults round as well.
> - I could watch a film with a friend.

Write down your ideas here (remember to include ridiculous ideas as well to get the ideas flowing):

Step 3: Look at the pros and cons of each possible activity

Example: Looking at Julia's ideas

Ideas from Step 2	Pros	Cons
First a crazy idea – I could fly everyone out to a desert island!	It would be nice. Maybe we could have an all-inclusive with 24-hour baby care!	I don't have the money. That's one of those whacky ideas to start off with!
I could invite some friends for lunch	That would be fun. But where would Ben go? Even with Ben around it would be nice to see some friends	What if Ben cried all the time? He may be awake. It wouldn't be much of a rest for me
I could invite one or two friends for a walk in the park	Getting out might be good fun	What if it rained? What if Ben is sick or very noisy?
I could do something with others and leave Ben with someone like mum	I'd have some free time – and could chat and enjoy time with others	Mum is pretty busy herself. I'd have to make sure she was okay about this and not stay away too long
I could have a children's party and invite all the adults round as well	Hmm. Might be good to chat to the adults	I'm not at all sure – with all those children we'd never get a chance to talk!
I could watch a film with a friend(s)	I used to like going to films and haven't been out anywhere for a long time. I'd love to see that new romantic comedy	Again, I couldn't take Ben – it's too risky, he'd be noisy. Might someone be able to look after him for two to three hours?

Write down your list of possible helpful activities into the following table, along with the pros and cons of each suggestion.

My suggestions from Step 2	Pros (advantages)	Cons (disadvantages)

Step 4: Choose one of the activities

From your list in Step 3, pick an activity that is realistic and likely to give you a boost. Choose something that gets you moving in the right direction. This should be small enough to be possible, but big enough to move you forwards. Sometimes it's helpful to think of this as many small steps that will help you move forwards.

Example: Julia's first step

Julia decides to ask her friends Emma and Sally round for lunch (her second idea). She also decides to ask her mother to look after Ben while they are round (her fourth idea).

Write down what you are going to try first here: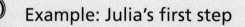

To check out if this helpful activity is the right thing to do, answer these **Questions for effective change**:

Q Will it be *useful* for changing how you are?

Yes ☐   No ☐

Q Is it a *clear* activity so that you will know when you have done it?

Yes ☐   No ☐

Q Is it something that is realistic, practical and achievable?

Yes ☐   No ☐

If you answered 'Yes' to all the three questions your chosen activity will be right to start with. If you answered 'No', go back to your list and look again carefully at what you can do.

Step 5: Plan the steps needed to do your helpful activity

You need to plan **what** you are going to do and **when** you are going to do it.

 Example: Julia's plan

Julia phones her mother and agrees two possible times next week when her mum can look after Ben. She then phones her two friends. They have a nice catch-up on the phone while Ben sleeps in the early evening. She agrees that they will meet next Tuesday for lunch at Emma's house – and then go for a walk in the park if the weather's nice. Otherwise they will stay at Emma's house.

Julia plans to drop Ben off at her mum's at 12, and then walk to Emma's for 12.30. She will take her umbrella if the weather forecast says it may rain. Julia also thinks through what she will do, if for whatever reason someone is ill. She will phone round and they'd try to plan it for some other time.

Now write down your plan. Make it very clear so that you know what you are going to do, and when you are going to do it. Also think about anything that may block your plan and how you will unblock it.

Now answer these **Questions for effective change**:

Does your plan:

- Include an activity that is realistic, practical and achievable?

  Yes ☐   No ☐

- Make clear what you are going to do and when you are going to do it?

  Yes ☐   No ☐

- Include what you will do if something blocks your plan?

  Yes ☐   No ☐

- Help you learn useful things even if it doesn't work out perfectly?

  Yes ☐   No ☐

If you have answered 'No' to any question, try to change the plan until you answer 'Yes' to all the questions.

What if your plan doesn't work out? Write down what you could do instead here:

Remember, large changes can be achieved by taking things one step at a time. Don't push yourself too hard or choose something to do that is too big or too fast.

Step 6: Now carry out your planned activity

> ### Example: Julia tries her plan
>
> Julia is about to set off to her mum's flat when suddenly Ben is sick over Julia's top. Julia is about to burst into tears when she thinks, 'Well I didn't predict that'. She puts Ben down on his mat and races upstairs to try to sponge the mess off. The top looks like it will need cleaning. She is tempted just to phone round and cancel when she decides – 'No, I'm going to go anyway'. She quickly changes her top and sets off.
>
> Julia drops Ben at her mother's and then has a nice time at Emma's with her and Sally. The three friends have a nice walk in the park as well. Julia feels a sense of happiness, achievement and also a real sense of closeness to her friends. They agree to meet again at her house next week.

Now carry out your planned activity ...

Pay attention to any thoughts and fears about what will happen before, during and after you have completed your plan. Write any thoughts/fears you noticed here:

Try to do your plan anyway. Good luck!

Step 7: Review what you have learned

> ## Example: Julia reviews her plan
>
> That was great. It would have been so easy for me to cancel. When Ben was sick over me I almost died! I was so upset and so down. But I handled it well – I put him down on his mat, and chose to get changed and go anyway. I'm so pleased I did. That was a real pick me up.
>
> I really enjoyed the lunch. And it was good to get outside in the park as well without the pram, just chatting away and feeling the sun on my face. I'm looking forward to next week.

Now write down your review here:

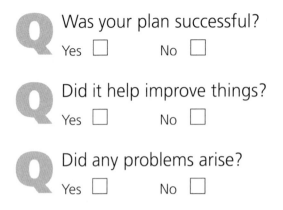

Q Was your plan successful?
Yes ☐   No ☐

Q Did it help improve things?
Yes ☐   No ☐

Q Did any problems arise?
Yes ☐   No ☐

What have you learned from doing this?

Write down any helpful lessons or information you have learned from what happened. If things didn't go quite as you hoped, try to learn from what happened.

 How could you make things different during your next attempt to do a helpful activity?

 Were you too ambitious or unrealistic in choosing the target you did?

If you noticed problems with your plan

Choosing realistic targets for change is important. Did you pick on too big an activity that you couldn't do in the time you had? Sometimes when you're trying to solve a problem in a planned way, it may get blocked by something unexpected. Perhaps something didn't happen as you planned, or someone reacted in an unexpected way? Still, try to learn from what happened.

Planning the next steps

Now that you have reviewed how your first step went, the next step is to plan another change to build on this first one. You need to think about your **short-term, medium-term** and **longer-term** targets. This means, where you want to be in a few weeks time (short term), in a few months time (long term) or in a year's time (long term)?

Key point

You will need to slowly build on what you have done in a step-by-step way.

You can choose to:

● Repeat the same plan you have just completed.

● Move it on a bit more.

● Practise another helpful behaviour.

Remember to think about the pros and cons of each choice for you.

Tips for choosing the next helpful behaviour

Create your own clear plan that will move things forward one step at a time.

Do:

● Be realistic. Plan to try **only** one or two activities over the next week.

● Make sure your **action plan** includes breaking down your chosen activity into smaller steps if it doesn't seem realistic and practical to do all together.

● Write down your plan in detail so you have a clear idea of what you will do and have predicted things that may block your plan from happening.

Don't:

● Try to plan too big an activity all at once.

● Be negative and think, 'I can't do anything, what's the point, it's a waste of time'. Experiment to find out if this negative thinking is right or helpful.

Write down your next steps here:

Key point

Stick to a plan, learn from what happens and make changes in a step-by-step way. You will grow in confidence and be able to respond helpfully when facing problems in the future.

Summary

In this workbook you have:

- Learned about helpful things you can do that will give you a boost.

- Tried a way of planning that works well to build helpful activities into your life.

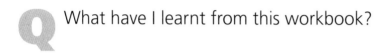 What have I learnt from this workbook?

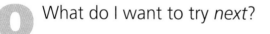 What do I want to try *next*?

Putting what you have learned into practice

Put what you have learned into practice over the next few weeks. Plan out what to do at a pace that is right for you. Build changes one step at a time.

My notes

Overcoming Postnatal Depression
A Five Areas Approach

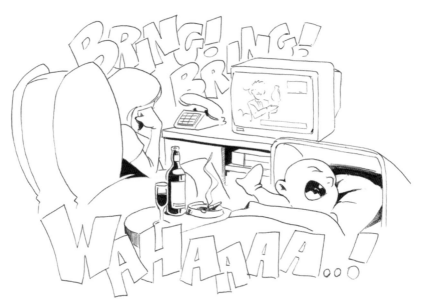

Unhelpful things you do

www.livinglifetothefull.com
www.fiveareas.com

Dr Chris Williams, Dr Roch Cantwell and Karen Robertson

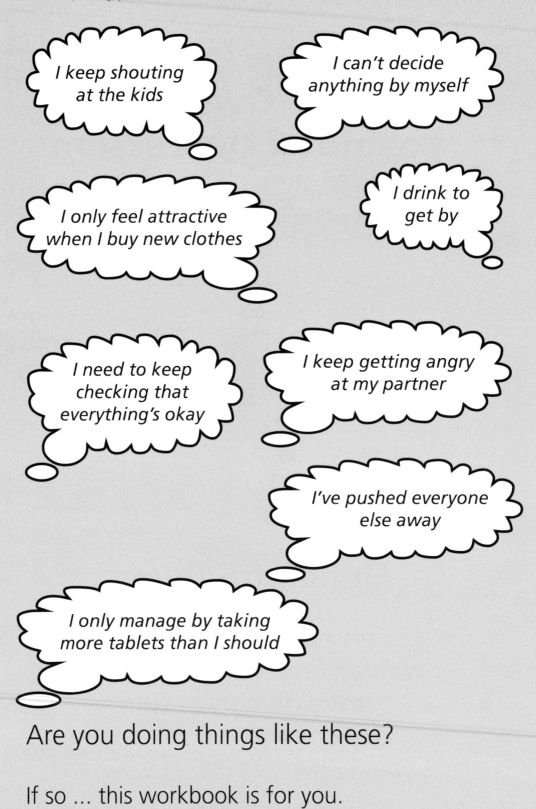

Are you doing things like these?

If so ... this workbook is for you.

> # In this workbook you will:
>
> - Find out about how some things can make you feel worse.
> - Learn some helpful ways to tackle unhelpful behaviours.
> - Make a clear plan to reduce an unhelpful behaviour.
> - Plan some next steps to build on this.

Helpful and unhelpful behaviours

When somebody feels distressed, it is normal to try to do things to feel better. But their responses may be *helpful* or *unhelpful*. You can find out more about helpful behaviours in the workbook *Helpful things you do*.

Unhelpful behaviours

Some examples of common unhelpful behaviours are:

- Getting angry at others.
- Pushing people away.
- Drinking too much to block how you feel.

These behaviours are unhelpful because of the effect they have on everyone. Getting angry can end up with you feeling alone. This can prevent you getting the help and support the other person would otherwise have offered. So both you and they feel worse as a result.

Why do unhelpful behaviours happen?

People tend to do unhelpful things simply because these actions can make us feel better – **in the short term**. However, they can also backfire and create more problems. So eventually, they become part of your problem.

 Task

Look at the following list and tick any activity that you did in the past few weeks. Many different unhelpful activities have been included in the list to help you to think about the unhelpful things that could be happening in your life.

Checklist: Identifying your unhelpful behaviour

As a result of how you feel, do you:	Tick here if you have noticed this – even if just sometimes
Eat too much to block how you feel ('comfort eating') or eat so much that this becomes a 'binge'?	☐
Feel anxious and aware all the time about symptoms of ill health?	☐
If you have this problem, you should discuss with your doctor whether you have symptoms of health anxiety or a physical cause of your symptoms	☐
Make impulsive decisions about important things?	☐
For example, resigning from a job without really thinking through the consequences	
Check your baby's health all the time?	☐
Set yourself up to fail?	☐
Try to spend your way out of how you feel by going shopping ('retail therapy')?	☐
Become very demanding or excessively seek reassurance from others?	☐
Watch television such as soaps or browse the internet, etc. to block how you feel – and act as a substitute for other relationships around you?	☐
Look to others to make decisions or sort out problems for you?	☐
Drink too much or use illegal drugs or prescribed medication to block how you feel or improve how you sleep, etc.?	☐
Set yourself up to be rejected by others?	☐
Throw yourself into doing things so that you are too busy to think about emotional or relationship issues?	☐
Not let others help with baby care	☐

As a result of how you feel, do you:	Tick here if you have noticed this – even if just sometimes
Look to others to do all the baby care	☐
Push others away by being verbally or physically rude to them?	☐
Deliberately harm yourself to block how you feel?	☐
Take risks, for example cross the road without looking, or gamble using money you don't have?	☐
Check, clean or feel compelled to do things a set number of times or in exactly the 'correct' order so as to make things 'right'?	☐
Or do you spend a lot of time deliberately thinking 'good' thoughts to make things feel 'right' or counting good things you've done?	☐
If so, you should see your doctor to discuss whether you may have a condition called obsessive-compulsive disorder	
Avoid having sex with your partner because you aren't interested, or because you feel unattractive or angry	☐

Write in any other unhelpful behaviours you've noticed yourself doing here:

Now think back on your answers.

Q Are some of your behaviours unhelpful in the short-term or longer-term either for you or for others?

Yes ☐   No ☐   Sometimes ☐

Here are some examples of exactly how these behaviours can backfire.

Example: Helen's temper

Helen had her son Jamie two years ago. Ever since then she has been suffering from postnatal depression. Everything seems hard, and Helen has noticed she quickly flies off the handle. She has been shouting at her partner Steve, and also at Jamie. At the time she sees the shouting as letting off steam, but afterwards she feels guilty and even more down.

Once or twice Helen has felt like hitting Jamie but instead has put him down safely and left the room. Steve is increasingly worried about Helen, but her temper outbursts are beginning to make him feel angry himself – at what he sees as unfair criticism. They are drifting apart as a couple as a result, and Steve is spending less time in the house.

Key point

Both *helpful* and *unhelpful* behaviours make you feel better in the short term. But the key difference between them is that in the longer-term **unhelpful behaviours backfire**. They worsen how you or others feel. So they become part of your problem. The good news is that if this applies to you, you can make changes.

Think about any behaviours you do that are unhelpful.

Q What effect do they have on you and those around you, in the short and longer term?

Choose just one example and write down its effect.

Effect on me:

Effect on others:

Unhelpful support from other people

Some people may offer 'helpful advice' all the time and want to do **everything** for you. There can be many reasons for this such as being concerned about you, friendship or love. Sometimes it may be because the other person feels anxious or even guilty about your low mood. Whatever the cause, when others offer too much help and want to do everything for us, their actions can backfire:

- You may feel suffocated and frustrated.
- You may feel treated like a child.
- Irritation may build up and upset both you and the other person.
- Their support may make you feel less confident.

Key point

When trying to cope with low mood it's important that you continue to do as many things as you are able to do. If others take over too much responsibility from you, the danger is that this will damage your confidence.

But there's good news. Discovering that unhelpful behaviours are part of what's keeping you feeling low, means that you have now identified something you can change. By working through the seven steps described below you can learn an approach that will help you change any unhelpful behaviour.

Overcoming your own unhelpful behaviour

Step 1: Identify and clearly define the unhelpful behaviour

Did you tick several boxes in the checklist on pages 230–231? The first thing to do is to choose just one unhelpful behaviour to change.

Example: Helen's temper

Helen decides she wants to works on her losing her temper.

Choosing a first target

Now, write down one single unhelpful behaviour that you want to change here:

Be a detective

The next thing is to do some research on your behaviour. First, record your unhelpful behaviour over several days. Make a written note of:

- When it occurs.
- How much and how often you do it (for example, how much you drink, how many times you've sought reassurance, etc.).
- How long it lasts for.

Use the **diary** at the end of this workbook to help you understand more about your unhelpful behaviour. Try to work out what it may be that affects how you respond at the time. For example:

● The time of day.

● Who you are with and how they responded.

● How you feel emotionally.

● What went through your mind.

● Whether you have slept well the night before.

● How you felt emotionally and physically at the time.

● Any other things you tend to do to cope or escape.

● And anything else that seems to help explain your reaction.

Check point: Is your target a realistic target? Answer the **Questions for change** to find out:

 Is your target:

● Clear and realistic and something that you can tackle over the next week or two?

Yes ☐   No ☐

● Not so scary that you can't face doing it?

Yes ☐   No ☐

● Still helping you move forwards?

Yes ☐   No ☐

Key point

Sometimes you need to make sure that your first target really is a small, focused problem so that you can tackle it in one step.

Now use your diary to decide if you need to break down the unhelpful behaviour into smaller steps that you can target one at a time.

 Do you need to break it down into a number of smaller more achievable targets?

Yes ☐   No ☐

If you answered 'Yes', then please go straight to Step 2. If you answered 'No', then keep reading about how to make sure you've chosen a realistic first target and write it here again.

Now write down your clear first step in tackling your target:

Example: Helen breaks her target into smaller steps

Helen keeps a record of when she gets angry and loses her temper. She realises that several things affect this. It's often when:

- She has slept poorly.
- When Jamie comes asking to play.
- Steve is at the pub.

Helen realises there are three separate things here she could work on. But she decides as a first step to focus on how she can respond when Jamie comes to play.

My clear first step is:

Remember this should be a small, focused problem you can tackle in one step.

Step 2: Think up as many solutions as possible to stop your unhelpful behaviour

Now you need to come up with as many ideas as possible. From among them you should be able to identity a realistic, practical and achievable solution.

Try to **think broadly**. Include completely whacky ideas in your list as well, even if you wouldn't choose to do them. Here are some useful questions to help you to think up possible solutions:

- What advice would you give a friend who was trying to do the same thing? (Sometimes it's easier to think of solutions for others than for yourself.)
- What *ridiculous* solutions can you include as well as more sensible ones?
- What helpful ideas would others (for example, your family, friends or colleagues at work) suggest?
- What approaches have you tried in the past in similar circumstances?

Key point

If you feel stuck, sometimes doing this task with someone you trust can be helpful.

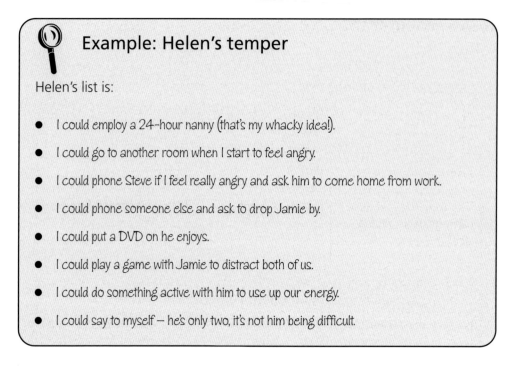

Example: Helen's temper

Helen's list is:

- I could employ a 24-hour nanny (that's my whacky idea!).
- I could go to another room when I start to feel angry.
- I could phone Steve if I feel really angry and ask him to come home from work.
- I could phone someone else and ask to drop Jamie by.
- I could put a DVD on he enjoys.
- I could play a game with Jamie to distract both of us.
- I could do something active with him to use up our energy.
- I could say to myself – he's only two, it's not him being difficult.

Now write down your list (including ridiculous ideas at first) here:

Step 3: Look at the pros and cons of each possible solution

Example: Helen's list of pros and cons

Ideas	Pros	Cons
I could employ a 24-hour nanny (that's my whacky idea!)	It would be great	We can't afford it. I'm not so sure how great it would feel. I want to see him grow up myself
I could go to another room when I start to feel angry	It would mean I could avoid upsetting him	He would probably follow me
I could phone Steve if I feel really angry and ask him to come home from work	It would be great if he could help more sometimes when I really need him	He's got a job commitment. I think if I felt near to hitting Jamie I'd phone him – but otherwise it's not fair on him
I could phone someone else and ask to drop Jamie by	I've several friends who help would understand and help if they could	I could probably only ask a few times. It wouldn't be a very good first response every time
I could put a DVD on he enjoys	He loves his builder's DVD. He always settles down when he watches it	I don't like the idea of him watching telly too much
I could play a game with Jamie to distract both of us	He loves building block games and then knocking the blocks over	I may not always be able to just stop doing things. This would work well though if there's time
I could do something active with him to use up our energy	We could have some small races. He enjoys that	I've never been one for running around. I'd get out of puff!
I could say to myself – he's only two, it's not him being difficult	I know it's true. I need to keep reminding myself of this	This might not be enough. If things have built up I think I need to do something to distract myself. Thinking differently doesn't seem to be enough for me

Write your list of ideas into the following table, along with the pros and cons of each suggestion.

My suggestions from Step 2	Pros (advantages)	Cons (disadvantages)

Step 4: Now choose one of the solutions

Choose a solution that is realistic and you think will be likely to succeed. Choose something that gets you moving in the right direction. It should be small enough to be possible, but big enough to move you forwards. Look at the list you made in Step 3 to help with this.

Example: Helen's choice

Based on Step 3, Helen decides next time she feels angry, she will play a game with Jamie to distract them both.

Write your choice here:

Now check your choice against some of the **Questions for effective change**:

Q Will it be useful for changing how you are?

Yes ☐   No ☐

Q Is it a specific task so that you will know when you have done it?

Yes ☐   No ☐

Q Is it realistic, practical and achievable?

Yes ☐   No ☐

Step 5: Plan the steps needed to carry it out

Write down the practical steps needed to carry out your plan. Try to be very clear in your plan so that you know **what** you are going to do, and **when** you are going to do it. Try to think through anything that could block you doing it, and have planned a way of tackling any problems that occur.

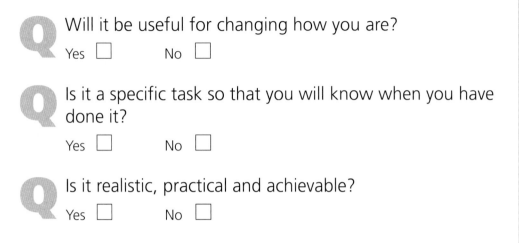

Example: Helen's plan

I'm going to watch out for times when I know I'm feeling hassled. Next time Jamie comes up to me wanting me to do something I'm going to do the reverse of sending him away and shouting. I'm going to slow down and stop. I'm going to choose to smile and say 'Jamie, let's build some bricks' and make a big deal over it. I know where the bricks are and this should work pretty much any time of day.

What could block things? Well, sometimes we really don't have time for a game – for example when we have to go to a doctor's appointment. If so I could explain it to him and maybe pretend we are going out together in the digger (the car).

Also if I just feel too hassled I'm going to have a back-up plan of putting on his favourite DVD. I'll give him a cuddle and pop his yellow builder's hat on. He loves builders. I'll then go and cool down somewhere else.

Now write down your plan here:

What if you think that there's something that may your block plan? Write down what you could do next to unblock it.

Remember that your plan needs to be a small step that you can achieve. Is it small and slow enough? If not go back and write it down again.

Now check your plan against the rest of the **Questions for effective change**:

Q Does your plan make clear what you are going to do and when you are going to do it?

Yes ☐   No ☐

Q Is it an activity that won't be easily blocked or prevented by practical problems?

Yes ☐   No ☐

Q Will it help me to learn useful things even if it doesn't work out perfectly?

Yes ☐   No ☐

Finally, before you carry on, try to think through what you will do if your initial plan doesn't work out.

Write your back-up plan here:

Step 6: Carry out the plan

Your task is to carry out this plan during the next week.

Here's where you find out if all that planning has helped you get a good plan.

Pay attention to any thoughts and fears about what will happen before, during and after you have completed your plan. Write any thoughts/fears you noticed here:

Try to do your plan anyway.

Good luck!

Step 7: Review the outcome

Example: Helen's review of her plan

Helen doesn't have too long to wait. She has a particularly busy day with friends round with their children in the morning. Then Jamie got over-tired and wouldn't settle for his afternoon sleep. As she tries to tidy the house, Jamie runs into the room with a big smile on his face and soil on his hands from a plant. Helen immediately feels angry and is about to shout when she stops, notices what is happening and decides instead to say 'Jamie, let's get you washed up. Do you want to play builders together?' Jamie is very excited, and as she cleans his hands Helen begins to settle down. They then spend 20 minutes building towers and knocking them down together.

Helen feels closer to Jamie than she has for some time and finds she enjoys it. Jamie certainly did. When Helen reviews the plan she realises it has helped her. Although she can't drop what she is doing every time, she has found that noticing her irritation, choosing not to get caught up in it by reacting immediately, and distracting her and Jamie onto something fun was good for both of them.

Now write down what happened in your plan here:

Q Was your plan successful?

Yes ☐   No ☐

Q Did it help improve things?

Yes ☐   No ☐

Q Did any problems arise?

Yes ☐   No ☐

What have you learned from doing this?

Write down any helpful lessons or information you have learned from what happened. If things didn't go quite as you hoped, try to learn from what happened.

How could you make things different during your next attempt to tackle an unhelpful behaviour?

 Were you too ambitious or unrealistic in choosing the target you did?

Planning the next steps

Now that you have reviewed how your first planned target went, the next step is to plan another change to build on this. You will need to slowly build on what you have done in a step-by-step way.

You have the choice to:

● Stop things now. You have achieved what you wanted to.

● Focus on the same problem area some more.

● Choose a new unhelpful behaviour to work on.

There are pros and cons of each of these choices. Think about these then make your choice.

Next, go on to consider your **short-term**, **medium-term** and **longer-term** targets.

> ## Example: Helen's short, medium and longer-term targets
>
> Helen's **short-term plan** over the next week or so: I want to keep practising playing with Jamie. I know I can't do that every time so I'll have playing his DVD as a back-up plan. If things build up too much I'll phone my friends and see if we can pop by.
>
> Helen's **medium-term plan** over the next few weeks: I want to start a discussion with Steve about him helping out more with the bedtime routine and the evening meal and helping tidying sometimes. That's going to need some planning! Maybe just one thing at a time – I don't want to over-burden the poor thing!
>
> Helen's **longer-term plan** over the next few months: I want to look at learning some ways of calming down when things build up. I also need to ask people for help when I need it. I think the *Being assertive* workbook might help that. Also the *Overcoming sleep problems* workbook because I know I feel far worse when I sleep badly.

Now it's your turn. In creating your plan:

Do:

- Plan to alter **only** one or two things over the next week.

- Plan to slowly alter things in a step-by-step way.

- Use the **questions for effective change** to check that the next step is always well planned.

- Write down your action plan in detail so that you know exactly what to do this week.

Don't:

- Try to alter too many things all at once.

- Choose something that is too hard a target to start with.

- Be negative and think '*Nothing can be done, it's a waste of time*'. Experiment to find out if this negative thinking is actually true.

Your short, medium and longer-term plans

Your short-term plan – what might you do over the next week or so? This is the next step you need to plan.

Your medium-term plan – what might you aim towards doing over the next few weeks – the next few steps?

Your longer-term plan – where do you want to be in a few months or so.

Remember to plan slow, steady changes. This will help you to rebuild your confidence, and increase your control over any unhelpful behaviours.

Summary

In this workbook you have:

- Found out about how some things we do make us feel worse.
- Learned some helpful ways to tackle unhelpful behaviours.
- Made a clear plan to reduce an unhelpful behaviour.

Q What have I learnt from this workbook?

Q What do I want to try *next*?

Putting what you have learned into practice

Can we encourage you with this plan? By taking small steps and keeping going large successes can be achieved. Don't try to solve every problem at once. Instead do things at a pace that is right for you. Build changes one step at a time.

My notes

My unhelpful behaviour diary

Day and date	Morning	Afternoon	Evening
Monday			
Tuesday			
Wednesday			
Thursday			
Friday			
Saturday			
Sunday			

Remember to record every time that you do the unhelpful behaviour.

Overcoming Postnatal Depression
A Five Areas Approach

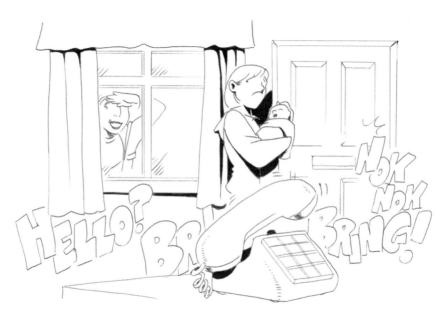

Anxiety and avoidance

www.livinglifetothefull.com
www.fiveareas.com

Dr Chris Williams, Dr Roch Cantwell and
Karen Robertson

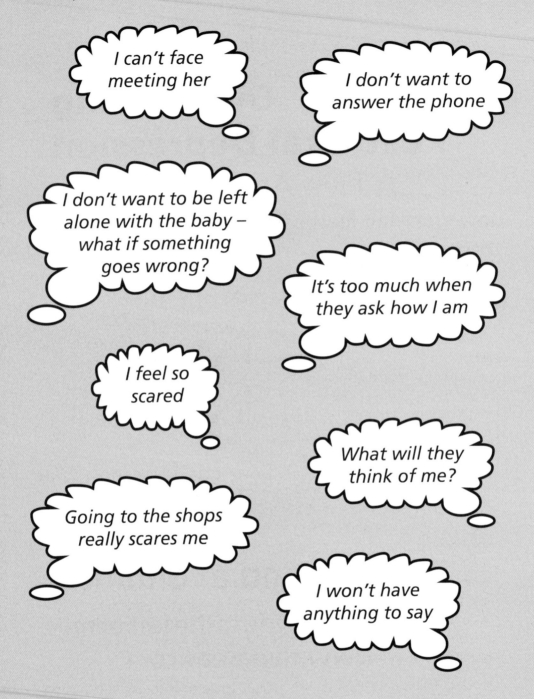

Are you feeling like this?

If so ... this workbook is for you.

In this workbook you will:

- Find out why you feel like avoiding things that seem scary.

- Learn how avoiding things can make your low mood worse.

- Make a clear plan to make slow, steady changes to tackle your avoidance.

- Plan some next steps to build on this.

How worrying fears affect how you feel

Have you noticed any change in your confidence since you started feeling low? Often, being in a low mood makes your confidence drop too and you start to feel more anxious about things.

Have you been worrying about things and feeling you can't cope, or that things will go wrong? Sometimes when you have a low mood, these fears can build up. And if your anxiety reaches a very high level (panic) you may want to leave or escape from the situation that's making you feel like this.

Here's how panic and high levels of anxiety can affect you in five key areas of your life:

1. **Area 1: People and events.** Sometimes people can become anxious about being in social situations. For example, you may be anxious about having a one-to-one conversation, or about how you behave in a group or when you have to give a presentation (such as giving a talk). You may think new challenges can seem scary. For example, picking up your baby and washing them for the first time. Or putting on a nappy, breastfeeding them, giving them their first bath, or going along to the parent and toddler group for the first time. There are so many things that can make you feel anxious. Whether you feel able to cope with these different situations is affected by the other areas of your life. You may also feel overwhelmed by other problems you currently face.

2. **Area 2: Thinking.** When you are feeling a little anxious you tend to get worrying thoughts about the past, what's going on now, or you may have concerns about the future. When people worry, they tend to go over things again and again without actually sorting out the things they are worried about. All this worry can turn you in on yourself. And it affects how you feel and what you do (see Areas 3, 4 and 5 below). Sometimes when you are extremely anxious, you may become very scared – predicting that the very

worst, most awful thing will happen. This is called 'catastrophic thinking' (for more about this style of thinking see the *Noticing and changing extreme and unhelpful thinking* workbook).

3. **Area 3: Feelings (emotions)**. When you are worried somewhat, you feel anxious but you can cope with it. But if you begin to feel very scared you can become panicky and terrified. Sometimes all sorts of other emotions occur. For example, you may feel irritable and angry at things you would usually cope with.

4. **Area 4: Altered physical symptoms**. When you feel scared your body also reacts. When you are feeling a little anxious, you may notice feelings of tension, or you may feel fidgety or find it hard to get off to sleep. When you are feeling even more anxious, you are likely to notice even stronger physical symptoms. You may feel hot or sweaty, shaky or cold, your heart rate goes up and you take rapid shallow breaths, and you may feel dizzy or faint. You may also have an urge to go to the toilet or feel sick. All of these are common and normal things that happen to everyone at times of anxiety.

Q Why do you have these physical symptoms when you feel panicky?

Your body reacts to extreme and unhelpful frightening thoughts just as it would to a physical danger. The **fight or flight adrenaline response** creates all of the symptoms described above. Your heart rate and breathing both speed up so that your muscles are ready to react to defend yourself or run away. This is very useful when the danger is real. Think about a time when you may have had a sudden shock. Perhaps you stepped into the road when a car was coming and didn't realise it until you heard the car's horn. In such a situation, your body releases adrenaline – which makes your heart beat faster. The fight or flight adrenaline response causes you to pay particular attention to anything around you that may cause you harm. You may have other physical

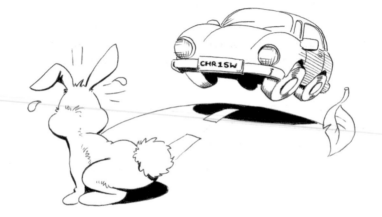

responses, such as feeling sweaty or restless and tense. Blood is pumped faster round your body so that your muscles are ready to react. And your breathing may speed up to allow more oxygen to get to your muscles so again you are ready to respond.

Sometimes when you continue to breathe rapidly for long enough you get in a state of anxious over-breathing – this is called *hyperventilation*.

You can find out more about these sorts of symptoms and the fight or flight adrenaline response in the companion book in this series *Overcoming Anxiety: A Five Areas Approach* by Chris Williams.

Key point

Feelings of anxiety are common and a normal reaction to fear. They are unpleasant but not dangerous.

5. **Area 5: Altered behaviours**. Other workbooks in this course talk about the *Helpful things you do* and *Unhelpful things you do*, and also *Doing things that boost how you feel*. This workbook focuses on one of the most common things that people do when you feel anxious – **avoiding things**.

Avoidance and its effect on you

Some of the things people start avoiding when they're feeling low are:

- **Meeting other people or going to particular places or situations** where you think you will feel worse. For example, people who fear feeling worse in shops (sometimes called agoraphobia) will avoid going into larger, busier shops. Similarly, someone who is very nervous about talking to others will try hard to avoid such situations, such as going to a new mums group. Or they **may try to arrive late** and then leave early – or avoid talking to people there. Does that sound like you?

- **Activities you are scared of**. You may look to others to help you with particular tasks or decisions. So you may decide in your mind that you can't do a particular activity. For example, some mothers worry about bathing their baby in case they drop or hurt them. Or you may avoid playing with your baby in case you think they aren't having fun.

- **Your physical health**. Sometimes you may have worries about how your activities are affecting your physical health. This is sensible if there is a clear reason to limit things – for example, you may have had a caesarean or you have a condition such as asthma. But sometimes we can overdo it. For example, someone with exercise-induced asthma may become so anxious about another attack that they avoid **any** activity. They lose confidence in their ability to do things 'just in case' it makes them feel worse. This doesn't mean all physical symptoms are caused by feeling low or anxious. If you notice new or worsening physical symptoms these need to be checked out by a doctor. But it's worth knowing that depression can often raise all sorts of fears about your physical health, and to think about whether this may be affecting you.

Whatever the cause, when you try to avoid things it adds to your problems by sapping your confidence. Also, avoidance tends to affect more and more things over time. That's why it's important to stop it taking over.

Key point

The problem with avoidance is that it teaches you that the **only** way to deal with a difficult situation is by avoiding it. This worsens your anxiety and saps your confidence. In fact often the best way of tackling your fears is to face them in a planned, step-by-step way. This also helps you test out whether your fears are actually true.

Things I avoid doing

Ask yourself 'What have I stopped or avoided doing because of my worries/concerns?' Remember that at times the avoidance can be quite **subtle**. For example, choosing to go to the shops at a time you know they are quiet, and then rushing through the shopping as quickly as possible.

Write down any examples of avoidance you may have noticed:

Now answer the following questions:

Q Are you avoiding things because they feel too difficult or scary?

Yes ☐   No ☐   Sometimes ☐

Q Has this reduced your confidence in things and led to a more restricted life?

Yes ☐   No ☐   Sometimes ☐

Q Overall has this worsened how you feel?

Yes ☐   No ☐   Sometimes ☐

If you have answered 'Yes' or 'Sometimes' to all three questions, then avoidance is causing problems for you.

Key point

The good news is that once you have noticed that you are avoiding things, you can begin to start tackling it.

Seven steps to tackling avoidance

You may have tried to stop avoiding things before. But unless you have a clear plan and stick to it, change will be hard to make. Making one change at a time is the key thing to help you move forwards. This may mean choosing at first **not** to focus on other areas.

By setting targets you can focus on how to make the changes needed to get better. To do this, you need to decide your:

- **Short-term** targets – these are the changes you can make today, tomorrow and the next week.

- **Medium-term** targets – these are the changes to be put in place over the next few weeks.

- **Long-term** targets – this is where you want to be in six months or a year.

By working through the seven steps below you can learn how to plan clear ways of overcoming avoidance. The aim is to slowly plan **specific** activities to boost your confidence and tackle avoidance. The good news is that you plan this one step at a time so it never seems too much or too scary.

Step 1: Identify and clearly define your problem

The following table lists the activities that are commonly avoided when you have low mood or depression. You will probably have noticed avoiding at least some of these activities.

Checklist: Identifying your patterns of worsening avoidance

As a result of how you feel are you:	Tick here if you have noticed this – even if just sometimes
Avoiding specific situations, objects, places or people because of fears about what harm might result?	☐
For example, shops, heights, spiders, meeting or talking to people, etc.	☐
Putting off dealing with important practical problems (both large and small)?	☐
For example, paying a cheque you received when your child was born into a Child Trust Fund	
Not really being honest with others?	☐
For example, saying yes when you really mean no or by not saying things that you really want to?	
Trying hard to avoid situations that bring about upsetting thoughts/memories?	☐
Avoiding physical activity or exercise that you should be able to do, because you have lots of worries about your physical health?	☐
Avoiding opening or replying to letters or bills?	☐
Sleeping in to avoid doing things or meeting people?	☐
Looking to others to sort things out for you?	☐
Avoiding answering the phone, or the door when people visit?	☐
Avoiding having sex?	☐

As a result of how you feel are you:	Tick here if you have noticed this – even if just sometimes
Avoiding talking to others face to face?	☐
Avoiding being with others in crowded or hot places, or busy and large shops?	☐
Avoiding going on buses, in cars, taxis, etc., or any places where it's hard to escape?	☐
Avoiding being left alone with your baby?	☐
Avoiding walking alone far from home?	☐
Stopping attending religious services, night classes or local pubs/clubs because it feels just too much to cope with at present?	☐

Write down any other activities you are avoiding here:

Example: Julia's avoidance

Ben is now a year old. But Julia has stopped going to playgroup with him because she's slowly felt more and more uneasy about going there. She felt very self-conscious when she was there and struggled to talk to the play leader or the other mothers. She would go red and feel she was stuttering.

Julia decides her first target in tackling avoidance will be to go back to the playgroup.

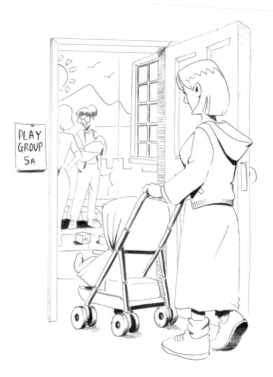

Choosing a first target

Now it's your turn. Use the list above to choose a single target that you will focus on to start with. This is particularly important if you have ticked several in the checklist. It isn't possible to work on all these areas at once. Instead you need to decide which **one** area to focus on to start with.

Write down one problem you want to work on here. (Remember that this should be a problem of avoidance.)

Be a detective

The next thing is to do some research on your avoidance. First, record in detail every time you avoid your chosen problem over several days. At the back of the workbook in the *My notes* section write down:

- What you avoid.

- When you avoid it.

- How much you do it (for example, don't go out, don't go to the shops, don't say hello – because of worries).

- How long it lasts for.

Try to understand more about your avoidance and why you tend to do it. Try to work out why you avoid or escape from things at that time such as:

- The time of day.

- Whether you slept well the night before.

- Who you were with and how they responded.

- How you felt emotionally.

- What went through your mind.

- How you felt emotionally and physically at the time.

- Any other things you did to try to cope or escape.

… And anything else that seems to help explain your reaction.

Write any key things you have learned here:

Check point: is your target a realistic target? Answer the **Questions for change** to find out:

 Is your target:

- Clear and realistic and something that you can tackle over the next week or two?

Yes ☐   No ☐

- Not so scary that you can't face doing it?

Yes ☐   No ☐

- Still helping you move forwards?

Yes ☐   No ☐

Key point

Sometimes you need to make sure that your first target really is a small, focused problem so that you can tackle it in one step.

Now use your notes to decide if you need to break down the avoidance behaviour into smaller steps that you can target one at a time.

Q **Do you need to break the avoidance down into a number of smaller more achievable targets?**

Yes ☐   No ☐

If you answered 'Yes', then please go straight to Step 2. If you answered 'No', then keep reading about how to make sure you've chosen a realistic first target and write it here again.

My clear first step is:

> ### Example: Julia breaks her target into smaller steps
>
> As Julia hasn't been going to playgroup at all she has very little information from her diary. But she has realised that she tries to avoid talking to people, even to the extent of crossing the road if she sees someone ahead she knows.
>
> Julia therefore decides to focus on something that would be a good first step towards going to playgroup – building confidence when she's talking to others. This is something that would help tackle a key problem for her – which is affecting whether she can go to playgroup.
>
> **Julia's target**: I'm going to focus on feeling more comfortable talking to others.

Step 2: Think up as many solutions as possible to achieve your initial target

Try to come up with as many ideas as possible. Try to **think broadly**. Include completely whacky ideas in your list as well, even if you wouldn't choose to do them. Here are some useful questions to help you to think up possible solutions:

- What advice would you give a friend who was trying to tackle the same problem?

- What ridiculous solutions can you include as well as more sensible ones?

- What helpful suggestions would others make?

- How could you look at the solutions facing you differently? What would you have said before you felt like this, or what might you say about the situation say in five years' time?

- What approaches have you tried in the past in similar circumstances?

Key point

If you feel stuck, sometimes doing this task with someone you trust can help.

> ### Example: Julia's ideas
>
> I could:
>
> - Pay an actor to be my friend and talk to me. I'd feel in charge then!
>
> - Start small – and build up my confidence on the phone.
>
> - Ask a friend to come round to chat so that I can practise talking again with someone I know likes me.
>
> - Just turn up at playgroup again.

Now write down as many possible options (including ridiculous ideas at first) for your own situation:

Step 3: Look at the pros and cons of each possible solution

Example: Julia's list of pros and cons

Idea	Pros (advantages)	Cons (disadvantages)
Pay an actor to be my friend and talk to me. I'd feel in charge then!	They'd be there all day. Maybe they could take me on a date too!	That's a crazy idea. But wouldn't it be great to have that much money
Start small – and build up my confidence on the phone	This is a small step which is great	I'm actually okay on the phone. It's more when I am with someone I start to go red and clam up
Ask a friend to come round to chat so that I can practise talking again with someone I know likes me	That sounds perfect. If it's someone I trust it wouldn't matter to me as much as someone who's not a friend. I could do that and I think it would help me build my confidence again	I might clam up. I don't think that's very likely though. I just need to plan a few conversation starters for if things go quiet. I can always play with Ben or ask about their children if I feel stuck so I think that's okay
Just turn up at playgroup again	Wouldn't that be great! I could go in and suddenly be confident all over again	It just doesn't seem that realistic. It's too big a step. I'd turn up and just sit alone in the corner feeling embarrassed. Or I'd leave and never go back

Write your own list of ideas into the following table, along with the pros and cons of each suggestion.

My suggestions from Step 2	Pros (advantages)	Cons (disadvantages)

Step 4: Now choose one of the solutions

Choose a solution that is a small step in the right direction and you think will be likely to succeed. Look at the list you made in Step 3 to help you with this.

The best way to tackle avoidance is to plan **steady, slow changes**. In this way, you can rebuild your confidence. The step should be small enough to be possible, but big enough to move you forwards.

Example: Julia's choice

Julia decides to ask a friend to come round to chat so that she can practise talking again with someone she knows she gets on with.

Key point

The first step you decide on should be something that helps you tackle your avoidance. If it seems scary, it shouldn't be so scary that you can't do it. You must be realistic in your choice so that the target doesn't appear impossible to do.

Write your choice here:

Now check your choice against some of the **Questions for effective change**.

Q Will your chosen step be useful for changing how you are?

Yes ☐   No ☐

Q Is it a specific task so that you will know when you've done it?

Yes ☐   No ☐

Q Is it realistic, practical and achievable?

Yes ☐   No ☐

If you answered 'Yes' to all three questions your chosen step should help start you off.

Step 5: Plan the steps needed to carry it out

You need to have a clear plan that will help you to decide exactly **what** you are going to do and **when** you are going to do it. **Write down** the steps needed to carry out your plan. This will help you to think what to do and also think of the possible problems that might arise. An important part of the planning process is also to try to think what could block the plan from happening or make it hard for you to follow it. That way you can think about how you would respond to keep your plan on track.

Example: Julia's plan

Julia phones her friend Emma who she knows from the local antenatal group. They have stayed in close touch since and have become good friends. Emma knows Julia has struggled with postnatal depression in the past and they can talk about most things. But Julia hasn't seen Emma for a few weeks and is a little nervous about how things will go. She therefore decides the following plan: 'Emma is coming by at 3 o'clock tomorrow. Ben should be awake by then. I'll get some scones in and I can heat them up with a cup of tea.'

Julia also tries to think of what might go wrong or cause her difficulties. She predicts she may feel uncomfortable about silences and therefore makes sure she plans a few questions to use to get things going if needed. She looks through the hints and tips for starting and keeping conversations going in the *Being assertive* workbook. And now she feels confident they will have things to talk about.

Now write down your plan here:

What if you think that there's something that may block your plan? Write down what you could do next to unblock it.

Now check your plan against the rest of the **Questions for effective change**:

Q Does it make clear what you are going to do and when you are going to do it?

Yes ☐   No ☐

Q Is it an activity that won't be easily blocked or prevented by practical problems?

Yes ☐   No ☐

Q Will it help you to learn useful things even if it doesn't work out perfectly?

Yes ☐   No ☐

Step 6: Carry out the plan

Your task is to carry this out during the next week.

As you get ready to put your plan into action be aware of worrying thoughts or fears. One of the best ways of checking how true unhelpful fears are is to act against them and see what happens.

Pay attention to any thoughts and fears you may have about what will happen before, during and after you have completed your plan. Write any thoughts/fears you noticed here:

If things seem just too scary, plan that you will carry out the plan anyway and see what happens. If things do seem too scary, then go back to Step 2 (your brainstorm) and pick something that is a less scary first step.

Good luck!

Step 7: Review the outcome

Example: Julia's review

Emma comes round as planned. She is a little late which makes Julia feel slightly more nervous. But when Emma arrives, Julia is too busy welcoming her and her son David to feel too anxious. They start off with her warming the scones which gives her something to do as they talk.

This seems to help a lot. Julia thinks that it would be useful to remember that doing something helps when she finally gets to playgroup. They have a lovely chat and Julia really enjoys it. Ben and David also seem happy together and there are no tantrums and only one set of tears.

Now write down your own review here:

Q Was your plan successful?
Yes ☐   No ☐

Q Did it help improve things?
Yes ☐   No ☐

Q Did any problems arise?
Yes ☐   No ☐

What have you learned from doing this?

Write down any helpful lessons or information you have learned from what happened. If things didn't go quite as you hoped, try to learn from what happened.

 How could you make things different during your next attempt to tackle your avoidance?

 Were you too ambitious in choosing the target you did?

Planning the next steps

Now that you have reviewed how your first planned target went, the next step is to plan another change to build on this. You will need to slowly build on what you have done in a step-by-step way.

You have the choice to:

- Stick with the target you have achieved.
- Focus on the same problem area and plan to keep working on this.
- Choose a new area to work on.

There are pros and cons of each of these choices. Think about these when you make your choice.

When you are making this decision, bear in mind that by practising the same step **again and again** over the next few weeks your confidence will grow. Your anxious fears will also get less and last for a shorter and shorter time.

This happens no matter what fear you try to tackle. Facing up to a fear causes it to slowly lose its effect on you. This is illustrated below.

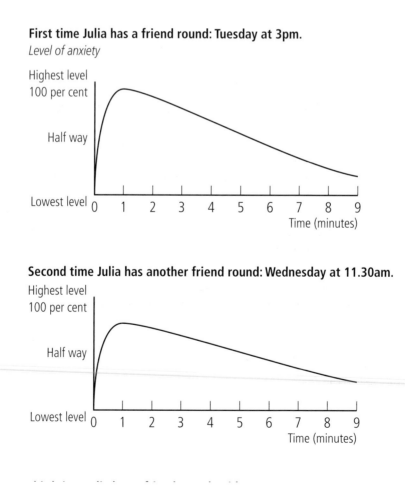

First time Julia has a friend round: Tuesday at 3pm.
Level of anxiety

Second time Julia has another friend round: Wednesday at 11.30am.

Third time Julia has a friend round: Friday at 3pm.

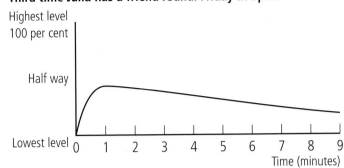

Key point

By facing up to your fears you can overcome them.

Next, think about your **short**, **medium** and **longer-term** targets.

Example: Julia's short, medium and longer term targets

Julia's **short-term plan** over the next week or so: I want to keep meeting up with friends, but to push myself by beginning to also meet several people together.

Julia's **medium-term plan** over the next few weeks: I want to build steps including meeting people I know less well, and in groups of two to three people. I also want to go along to playgroup by around six weeks time – perhaps with Emma to start with so there's a friendly face around. I'll also plan to start talking to people I don't know and saying hello with a big smile on my face and see what happens. Well I have paid for the term's fees – I need to get some value out of it!

Julia's **longer-term plan** over the next few months: I want to be able to go to playgroup and not even think about it. I want to be able to chat to anyone and not get worried about it.

Now it's your turn. In creating your plan:

Do:

- Plan to alter **only** one or two things over the next week.
- Plan to slowly alter things in a step-by-step way.
- Use the **questions for effective change** to check that the next step is always well planned.
- Write down your action plan in detail so that you know exactly what to do this week.

Don't:

- Try to alter too many things all at once.
- Choose something that is too hard a target to start with.
- Be negative and think 'It's a waste of time'. Experiment to find out if this negative thinking is actually true.

Your short, medium and long-term plans

Your short-term plan – what might you do over the next week or so? This is your next step you need to plan.

Your medium-term plan – what might you aim towards doing over the next few weeks – the next few steps?

Your longer-term plan – where do you want to be in a few months or so?

Remember to plan slow, steady changes. This will help you to re-build your confidence, as you tackle your avoidance. You'll also probably discover that facing fears is one of the best ways around of tackling your worries as well.

Summary

In this workbook you have:

- Found out why we avoid things that seem scary.
- Learned how avoiding things can make you feel worse.
- Made a clear plan to make slow, steady changes to tackle your avoidance.
- Planned some next steps to build on this.

 What have I learnt from this workbook?

 What do I want to try *next*?

Putting what you have learned into practice

The best way to make changes is by slow, steady steps. You're probably a bit fed up with reading this by now but it's true! If at any stage any step seems too much then go back to the drawing board (Step 2) and think up another smaller step you can cope with.

Good luck!

My notes

Overcoming
Postnatal Depression
A Five Areas Approach

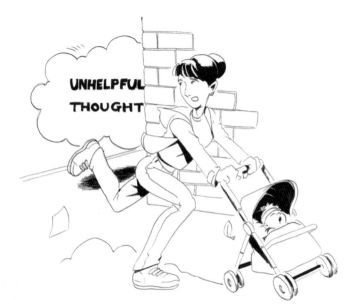

Noticing and changing extreme and unhelpful thinking

www.livinglifetothefull.com
www.fiveareas.com

Dr Chris Williams, Dr Roch Cantwell and
Karen Robertson

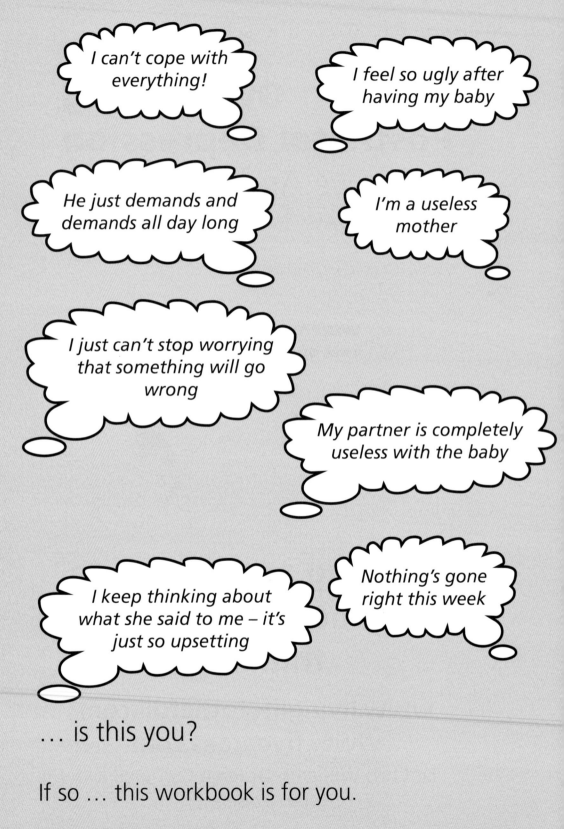

… is this you?

If so … this workbook is for you.

When you feel low or stressed you can:

- Feel anxious and fearful – these feelings make you tense and stressed.

- Have unhappy, negative thoughts – these can make you feel **low and sad** – even at times (like after having a baby) when you thought you'd be happy and excited.

- Have frustrated, angry thoughts about yourself, your situation and sometimes about others such as your baby, partner, friends and relatives.

You could have **all sorts of upsetting thoughts** about how you feel, your current situation and your future outlook.

In this workbook you will learn:

- How to recognise patterns of extreme and unhelpful thinking that worsen how you feel.

- How to change this sort of thinking so it's less upsetting.

The first step in changing unhelpful thinking is to start noticing how **common** it is in your life.

Key point

Frustration, anger, distress, shame, guilt and feeling down are often linked to unhelpful thinking.

Going through the checklist below will help you to recognise whether your thinking is unhelpful.

Checklist: The unhelpful thinking styles

Unhelpful thinking style	Some typical thoughts	Tick if you have noticed this thinking style recently – even if it's just sometimes
Being your own worst critic/bias against yourself	• I'm very self-critical • I overlook my strengths • I see myself as not coping • I don't recognise my achievements • I knew that would happen to me!	☐
Putting a negative slant on things (negative mental filter)	• I see things through dark-tinted glasses • I see the glass as being half empty rather than half full • Whatever I've done in the week it's never enough to give me a sense of achievement • I tend to focus on the bad side of everyday situations	☐
Having a gloomy view of the future (make negative predictions)	• I think that things will stay bad or get even worse • I tend to think that things will go wrong • If one thing goes wrong I often predict that everything will go wrong • I'm always looking for the next thing to fail	☐

Unhelpful thinking style	Some typical thoughts	Tick if you have noticed this thinking style recently – even if it's just sometimes
Jumping to the very worst conclusion (catastrophising)	● I tend to think that the very worst outcome will happen ● I often think that I will fail badly	☐
Having a negative view about how others see me (mind-reading)	● I mind-read what others think of me ● I often think that others don't like me or think badly of me without any reason for it	☐
Unfairly taking responsibility for things	● I think I should take the blame if things go wrong ● I feel guilty about things that aren't really my fault ● I think I'm responsible for everyone else	☐
Making extreme statements or rules	● I use the words *'always'* and *'never'* a lot ● If one bad thing happens to me I often say 'just typical' because it seems this *always* happens ● I make myself a lot of *'must'*, *'should'* *'ought'* or *'got to'* rules	☐

Almost everyone has these sorts of thoughts each and every day. This doesn't mean that:

● You think like this **all** the time.

● You have to notice **all** of the unhelpful thinking styles.

However, unhelpful thinking can affect how you feel.

Where do unhelpful thoughts come from?

While growing up, people learn to relate to others from their parents, teachers and friends. Some people also get influenced by other things such as television and magazines. You may read about how important it is to be a 'perfect' mother who smiles and irons, looks good, washes and cooks, and feels like having sex all the time. However, this image of perfect motherhood is impossible for anyone to live up to in the real world. Many mothers often mentally beat themselves up over things they *must/should/ought* to do, or over things they think they haven't done well. In doing so, you often overlook that actually you are doing a far better job than you are giving yourself credit for.

How does unhelpful thinking affect you?

Often we believe in these kinds of thoughts just because they '*feel*' true. And this is because of how you're feeling in yourself. But you can forget to check out how true these thoughts really are.

Usually when you notice these kinds of thoughts you may feel a little upset, but then quickly move on and carry on with life. But there are times when you're more prone to these thoughts and find them harder to dismiss. For example, when you have some problem you're finding hard to cope with or if you're distressed and worn down. It's quite normal for many new parents to have more of such thoughts because of the added demands of a new baby – especially when they aren't sleeping and are sometimes struggling to cope. At times like this, you may also dwell on such thoughts more than usual and find it harder to move on.

Remember that what you think can have a powerful effect on how you **feel** and what you **do**. So unhelpful thinking can lead to:

1 **Mood changes** – you may become more down, guilty, upset, anxious, ashamed, stressed or angry.

2 **Behaviour changes** – you may stop doing things or avoid doing things that seem scary. Or you end up reacting in ways that backfire, such as pushing others away or even drinking too much or using street drugs to cope.

Key point

The result is that unhelpful thinking styles worsen how you feel.

Task

The following table shows the links between thoughts, feelings and behaviour. You'll notice in the last column of the table there is a suggestion that stopping, thinking and reflecting (**before** getting carried away by the thought and just ending up feeling worse) could help you feel better.

Example: Dealing with unhelpful thinking

Situation	Unhelpful thinking style	Altered feelings	Altered behaviour
1. You are pushing the pram down the road and someone you know from the antenatal class walks past and says nothing. They don't smile or meet your eye – just walk by Thought: *There's poor Sam – she looks really distracted. I hope she's okay*	This is normal concern for others It isn't an unhelpful thinking style	Concern for Sam	You turn round and catch up with Sam to say hello. Sam looks a little surprised to begin with and says she didn't see you. You get chatting and have a really nice talk. At the end you both agree to meet for lunch after the shopping to catch up **Stop, think and reflect:** *I'm really pleased I spoke to her. It was nice to talk – and she seemed pleased too. She suggested we meet up for lunch which is good because it says to me that she wants to see me and enjoyed chatting*

2. You are pushing the pram down the road and someone you know from the antenatal class walks past and says nothing. They don't smile or meet your eye – just walk by	This is an unhelpful thinking style: mind-reading (that she don't like you); jumping to the worst conclusion; being your own worst critic; being biased against your own self	Low/down and upset; anxious in case you meet again	Feel so down you just go home; avoid Sam in future
Thought: *They don't like me*			**Stop, think and reflect**: *You never checked out that this was the real reason. Maybe Sam just didn't see you?*
3. You are at a supermarket checkout trying to pack your bags while your baby cries in the pram. You hear someone behind you tut as you pack the bags	This is an unhelpful thinking style: being your own worst critic, bias against yourself (blame yourself); mind-reading that they are irritated by your slowness and the crying	Anxiety; perhaps anger – 'how dare they – babies do cry you know!'	**If anxious**: maybe speed up packing – fumble and start to drop things. Make all sorts of apologies
Thought: *I'm being too slow. They're annoyed with me*			**If angry**: perhaps slow down the packing, stare at them or pass a sarcastic comment which backfires because you end up in an argument
			Stop, think and reflect: *Maybe they were tutting at something else. Maybe they'd forgotten to pick up the apples. Maybe their teeth don't fit!*

Key point

Thinking in these extreme ways means that you're only looking at part of the picture. Because of this, these thinking styles are often not true.

But what if my unhelpful thoughts are true?

Of course some of these thoughts can be true at times. For example, you are responsible for the safety and health of your baby. But others around you also have a part to play in this. Your health visitor, doctor and other health workers can help you, and offer useful advice and support. Family and friends may also be there to help with time, encouragement and practical support. So although you are responsible for most of the time, it becomes unhelpful if you focus on your negative thoughts and feel crushed by them.

The same is true for the other types of thoughts. Sometimes when we mind-read we are right – someone we know doesn't like us, or judge us well. But remember that when you feel low you worry too much about these things – and worry that almost everyone thinks this way without any reason for it to be true.

Being aware that most people are prone to thinking in this way at some time – and even more so when feeling low is important – because thinking like this is upsetting, wearing and affects how you live. The good news is it's possible to help get things back into balance.

Noticing extreme and unhelpful thinking

The next step is to practise ways of **noticing** extreme and unhelpful thinking. This is the first and most important step in beginning to change how you think. Once you can notice these patterns to your thinking you can step back and choose to make changes.

Here are some examples to help you try to see how extreme thinking may affect how you feel and what you do.

Example: Sally's unhelpful thinking (1)

Sally has had feelings of postnatal depression for the last nine months. She has tended to avoid meeting people because of low confidence. One day, someone from her antenatal group phones up to say they are all having lunch together. She says she will come along with her partner John and son Jack.

On the day Sally chooses to sit at the end of the table and avoids speaking to the others. She mind-reads that 'everyone else is a better mum than me' and this causes her to withdraw even more into herself.

Sally is also annoyed because John seems to be enjoying himself. She thinks 'He's more interested in them than me – he doesn't care'. She worries she doesn't have anything to say and that 'They won't be interested in speaking to me'. She feels physically tense too – with a rapid heartbeat and breathing (which happen when you feel anxiety) and feels sweaty. After the main course she turns to John and says that Jack is feeling unwell and needs to be taken home and goes to sit in the car, not saying goodbye to most of the group.

Sally's avoidance and mind-reading prevents her discovering that she would've really enjoyed things if she had started talking to others. Because of her fears she never did that. Instead she sat alone at the end of the table, cut off from the rest of them. Afterwards she is left 'feeling like a fool' for not having talked more to the others – and also angry at John. John is annoyed with her. He was enjoying catching up with people, and thinks that Sally has been rude for not saying goodbye. He feels frustrated and criticises her as a result. They both go to sleep that night angry at the other.

Sally's Five Areas thought review of a time when she felt worse (1)

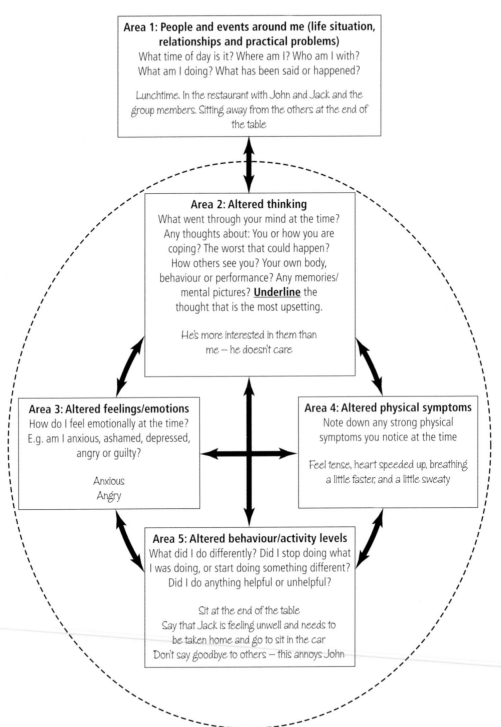

Area 1: People and events around me (life situation, relationships and practical problems)
What time of day is it? Where am I? Who am I with? What am I doing? What has been said or happened?

Lunchtime. In the restaurant with John and Jack and the group members. Sitting away from the others at the end of the table

Area 2: Altered thinking
What went through your mind at the time? Any thoughts about: You or how you are coping? The worst that could happen? How others see you? Your own body, behaviour or performance? Any memories/ mental pictures? **Underline** the thought that is the most upsetting.

He's more interested in them than me — he doesn't care

Area 3: Altered feelings/emotions
How do I feel emotionally at the time? E.g. am I anxious, ashamed, depressed, angry or guilty?

Anxious
Angry

Area 4: Altered physical symptoms
Note down any strong physical symptoms you notice at the time

Feel tense, heart speeded up, breathing a little faster, and a little sweaty

Area 5: Altered behaviour/activity levels
What did I do differently? Did I stop doing what I was doing, or start doing something different? Did I do anything helpful or unhelpful?

Sit at the end of the table
Say that Jack is feeling unwell and needs to be taken home and go to sit in the car
Don't say goodbye to others — this annoys John

Example: Sally's unhelpful thinking (2)

Sally's health visitor tells her how important it is for mothers to play with their baby. Sally immediately thinks 'She's saying I'm a bad mother because I'm not playing with Jack enough' and feels hurt, guilty and upset. She says to herself 'I'm useless' and also that 'I'm a bad influence on my baby'. She feels tense and restless. She becomes self-critical and thinks that John and her own parents are all better at playing with Jack than she is. As a result she looks to her parents to provide all the best playtime with Jack.

Here, Sally is being very self-critical (being her own worst critic/bias against herself), and she's overlooking the fact that she is the most important person in Jack's life. He spends more time with her than anyone else. She is interacting with him for lots of the day – quite the opposite of her thought 'I'm a bad influence on my baby'. By talking, washing, feeding, making eye contact, smiling and cuddling Jack she is helping his well-being and development.

Sally's Five Areas thought review of a time when she felt worse (2)

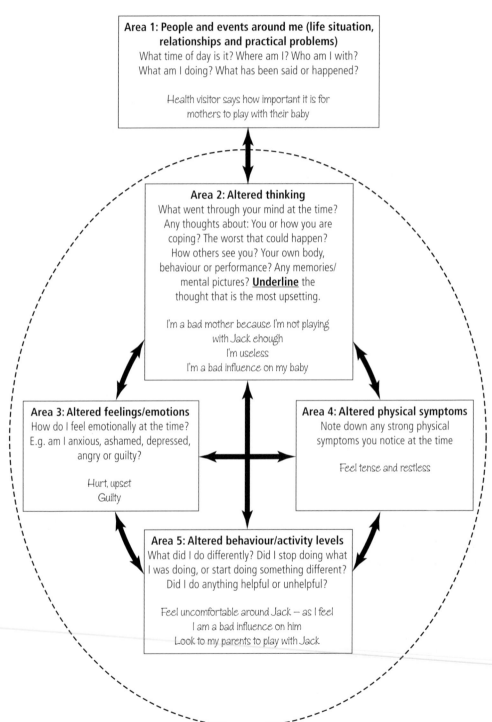

Area 1: People and events around me (life situation, relationships and practical problems)
What time of day is it? Where am I? Who am I with? What am I doing? What has been said or happened?

Health visitor says how important it is for mothers to play with their baby

Area 2: Altered thinking
What went through your mind at the time? Any thoughts about: You or how you are coping? The worst that could happen? How others see you? Your own body, behaviour or performance? Any memories/ mental pictures? <u>**Underline**</u> the thought that is the most upsetting.

I'm a bad mother because I'm not playing with Jack ehough
I'm useless
I'm a bad influence on my baby

Area 3: Altered feelings/emotions
How do I feel emotionally at the time? E.g. am I anxious, ashamed, depressed, angry or guilty?

Hurt, upset
Guilty

Area 4: Altered physical symptoms
Note down any strong physical symptoms you notice at the time

Feel tense and restless

Area 5: Altered behaviour/activity levels
What did I do differently? Did I stop doing what I was doing, or start doing something different? Did I do anything helpful or unhelpful?

Feel uncomfortable around Jack – as I feel I am a bad influence on him
Look to my parents to play with Jack

Completing your own thought review

Now let's look in detail at a particular time when you felt worse.

First, try to think yourself back into a situation in the past few days when your mood unhelpfully changed. To begin with **don't choose a time when you have felt very distressed**. Instead, pick an occasion when you noticed **some** not too severe upset, tension, symptoms, anger or guilt. Try to be as slow as you can when you think back through the situation, so that you're as accurate as you can be. If you can't think of such a situation carry on reading. If you can think of one go straight to the task at the bottom of this page.

What to do if you find it's hard to even think about the upsetting situation

Sometimes it can feel distressing going back over a time when you have felt worse. That's why it's important to choose a time that didn't make you feel too upset.

The idea here is to make you feel able to change such thoughts and to feel less distressed. Sometimes concerns, worries and fears can feel terrifying and too much to look at all in one go. So if you feel this way, the key is to practise this approach slowly, with less upsetting thoughts to begin with.

Start to notice the thoughts that link in with feeling **somewhat or moderately upset**. Work with these thoughts first, and use the rest of the workbook to practise changing these. You can slowly work up to more upsetting thoughts later when you are feeling more confident.

📌 Task

Now stop, think and reflect as you go through the five different areas that can be affected. Use the blank Five Areas diagram on page 299 to go through what you noticed in each of the Five Areas.

1. **People and events around you**: Think about the situation.

- Where were you?

- What time of day was it?

- Who else was there?

- What was said?

- What happened?

Write the answers in Box 1 of the Five Areas diagram.

2. **Altered thinking**:

- What went through your mind at the time?
- How did you see yourself?
- How were you coping (for example, did you have any bias against yourself, were you your own worst critic)?
- What did you think was the worst thing that could happen (were you expecting the worst, that is, catastrophic thinking)?
- How did you think others saw you (were you mind-reading)?
- What did you think about your own body and behaviour?
- Were there any painful memories from the past?
- Did you think up any images or pictures in your mind (images are another way of us thinking and also can have a powerful effect on how you feel)?

Write down any thoughts you notice into Box 2. **Underline** the most upsetting thought.

3. **Altered feelings**:

- How did you feel emotionally at the time?
- Were you anxious, ashamed, depressed, angry or guilty?

Write these things in Box 3.

4. **Altered physical symptoms**:

We often notice physical symptoms when we feel upset. You may have had many different physical feelings, for example:

- Muscle tension, jitteriness or pain in anxiety or anger.
- Other anxiety-related symptoms, such as a rapid heartbeat and rapid breathing, and feeling hot, sweaty and clammy.
- Poor concentration and feelings of low energy, pressure or even pain.

Write these things in Box 4.

5. Altered behaviour:

Remember that this can be:

- *Reduced activity* – you reduced or stopped doing what you had planned to do.
- *Avoidance or escape* – you suddenly felt anxious and avoided doing something or going somewhere or escaped from a situation without staying to see if the thing you fear really happened.
- *Unhelpful behaviours* – you tried to block how you felt by acting in ways that you thought would make you feel better. It may have done so then but backfired in the longer term.

Write these things in Box 5.

At the same time, did you also notice that there were other, more helpful, responses that you made?

Now look at how the different areas affect each other. Does what you think affect what you felt and what you did?

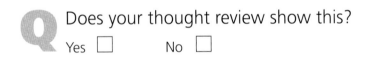

What you think ⟶ affects how you feel

What you think ⟶ affects what you do

Q Does your thought review show this?

Yes ☐   No ☐

There is another blank Five Areas assessment sheet at the end of this workbook. Copy this so you can practise this approach again and again. This is helpful because being aware of these patterns is an important step towards changing things.

At first, many people find it can be quite hard to notice their unhelpful thinking. But doing the thought review described here will help you to start noticing your thinking. Over time you'll find that this becomes easier to do. The best way of becoming aware of your thinking is to try to notice the times when your mood unhelpfully alters (for example at times when you feel upset), and then to ask 'What is going through my mind right now?'.

Remember, we all have all kinds of thoughts during the day. The thoughts we need to change are those that are:

- *Extreme* – that is, they show one of the unhelpful thinking styles.

And are also:

- *Unhelpful* – that is, they worsen how we feel and/or affect what we do.

My Five Areas thought review of a time when I felt worse

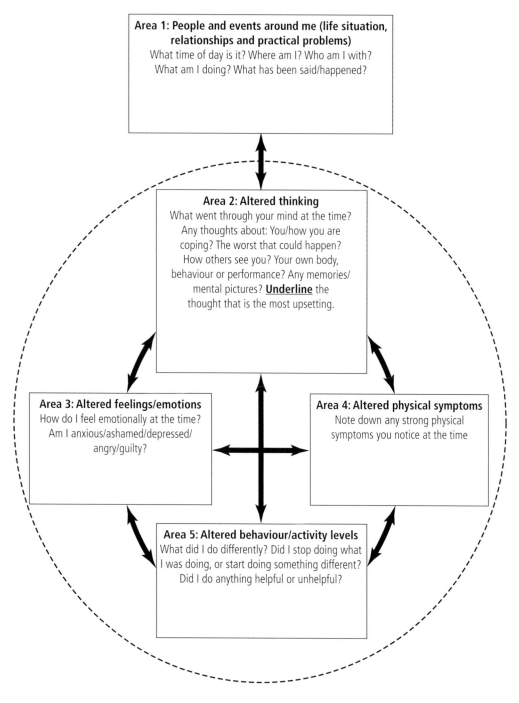

Area 1: People and events around me (life situation, relationships and practical problems)
What time of day is it? Where am I? Who am I with? What am I doing? What has been said/happened?

Area 2: Altered thinking
What went through your mind at the time? Any thoughts about: You/how you are coping? The worst that could happen? How others see you? Your own body, behaviour or performance? Any memories/mental pictures? **Underline** the thought that is the most upsetting.

Area 3: Altered feelings/emotions
How do I feel emotionally at the time? Am I anxious/ashamed/depressed/angry/guilty?

Area 4: Altered physical symptoms
Note down any strong physical symptoms you notice at the time

Area 5: Altered behaviour/activity levels
What did I do differently? Did I stop doing what I was doing, or start doing something different? Did I do anything helpful or unhelpful?

Hopefully, the Five Areas model has shown you that **what you think** about a situation or problem may **affect how you feel** physically and emotionally. It also may alter **what you do** (altered behaviour).

Changing our extreme and unhelpful thoughts

The following five steps are a **proved way of changing thoughts** that are extreme and unhelpful. You can use as many or as few of the following steps as you need. Just stop when you feel you can move on from the thought.

1. Label the thought as 'just one of those unhelpful thoughts', rather than 'the truth'.

2. Stop, think and reflect – don't get caught up in it.

3. Move on – act against it. Don't be put off from what you were going to do.

4. Respond by giving yourself a truly caring response.

5. Question the thought and ask yourself the seven thought challenge questions described later.

Let's look at each of the steps one at a time.

Step 1: Label the thought as 'just one of those unhelpful thoughts'

When you feel upset, use the list below to tick the unhelpful thinking patterns that are present at that time.

Unhelpful thinking style	Tick if your thought(s) showed this pattern at that time
Am I being my own worst critic? (Biased against yourself)	☐
Am I focusing on the bad in situations? (A negative mental filter)	☐
Am I making negative predictions about the future? (A gloomy view of the future)	☐
Am I jumping to the very worst conclusion? (Catastrophising)	☐
Am I second-guessing that others see me badly without checking if it's actually true? (Mind-reading)	☐
Am I *taking unfair responsibility* for things that aren't really my fault or taking all the blame?	☐
Am I using unhelpful *must* or *should* or *ought* or *got to* statements? (Making extreme statements or setting impossible standards)	☐

Key point

If the thought *doesn't* show one of the unhelpful thinking styles then you should stop here. Choose another time when you feel more upset, low, angry, anxious, ashamed or guilty and complete Step 1 again until you identify a thought that is an unhelpful thinking style. Then move on to Step 2.

Step 2: Stop, think and reflect – don't get caught up in it

Simply **noticing** that you're having an unhelpful thinking style can be a powerful way of getting rid of it.

- Label the upsetting thought as **just another** of those unhelpful or even silly thoughts. These are just a part of what happens when you are upset. It will go away and lose its power. It's part of distress – it's not the true picture. You could say to the thought: 'I've found you out – I'm not going to play that game again!'

- Allow the thought to **just be**. Don't allow yourself to get caught up in it. Don't bother trying to challenge the thought, or argue yourself out of it. Like a celebrity such thoughts love attention. They're just not worth your attention. Allow them to **just be**. Take a mental step back from the thought as if observing it from a distance. Move your mind on to other more helpful things – for example, the future, or recent things you have done well, or even better onto the task in hand.

Step 3: Move on – act against it. Don't be put off from what you were going to do

Unhelpful thinking worsens how you feel and unhelpfully alters what you do. The thought may push you to:

- Stop, reduce or avoid doing something you were going to do. This leads to a loss of pleasure and achievement. In the longer term it will restrict your life and undermine your confidence.

- Feel you must do something, like drinking, to cope. This is actually unhelpful. It ends up backfiring and worsening how you or others feel.

Make an **active choice** not to allow this to happen again. This often means acting against the thought. Choose to react helpfully rather than unhelpfully. Choose not to be bullied into changing what you do by the thought.

To stand up to the bully try these three dos and don'ts.

Do:

- **Keep doing** what you planned to do anyway. Stay active.
- **Face your fears**. Act against thoughts that tell you that things are too scary and you should avoid them. By taking a step-by-step approach you can overcome these fears. See the *Anxiety and avoidance* workbook.
- **Experiment**: If an extreme and unhelpful thought says don't do something – do it. If a thought says you won't enjoy going to that party, try going and see if you do.

Don't:

- Get pushed into not doing things by the thoughts.
- Let fear rule your life.
- Block how you feel with drink or even drugs or by seeking reassurance.

Step 4: Respond by giving yourself a truly caring response

(**Acknowledgement**: The concept of the 'compassionate mind' response was developed by Professor Paul Gilbert, among others.)

 What would someone who wholly and totally loved me say?

If a friend was troubled by a thought or worry, you would offer words of advice to soothe and encourage them. Imagine you have the best friend in the world. Someone who is totally on your side, totally loving and is totally caring. What words of advice and encouragement would they say to you? Write their caring advice here.

Think about this – choose to apply their words in your own situation. Trust what they say. Allow that trust to wash over you and take away the troubling thoughts. Speak them out loud in private, saying the words in a caring and compassionate way.

You might choose a close friend or relative. Or perhaps a famous person from literature, or, if you have a religious faith, someone from your scriptures. Whoever you choose you need to be aware that the response will be unconditionally positive, caring and supportive.

Example: Sally's caring thoughts

Sally chooses her Gran. She thinks back to what she would have said. These are words of support and love: 'You know we all love you Sally. People often lose their confidence when they feel upset. Don't worry that you didn't chat much with your friends this time – you did well getting out in the first place, it's not worth upsetting yourself about. You can always have a chat with them later. They'll be pleased to see you – just you see'.

Step 5: Question the thought and ask yourself the seven thought challenge questions

Our upsetting thoughts are often incorrect and untrue. Try to look at the thought in a logical way.

The questions you need to ask are:

- What would I tell a friend who said the same thing?
- Am I basing this on how I feel rather than on the facts?
- What would other people say?
- Am I looking at the whole picture?
- Does it really matter so much?
- What would I say about this looking back six months from the future?
- Do I apply one set of standards to myself and another to others?

Taking what works for you

When you use the approaches described above in this workbook, you'll probably find that some of the different responses are being more effective for you than some of the others. Build on the ones that work for you into your own reaction when you notice upsetting thoughts. Remember, practising will really help.

Also **discussing** your thoughts, fears and concerns with others can sometimes help you get them into a **different perspective** so they no longer seem upsetting.

Example: Sally changes her perspective

The next time Sally goes shopping and Jack cries she can say to herself 'No-one else is bothered, they all know and expect children will cry. It won't even matter in 10 minutes let alone six months. He'll settle down eventually, I'll just distract him with his toy.'

These thoughts help Sally change her perspective and feel less anxious. She carries on shopping rather than heading for the exit in embarrassment, apologising to people and rolling her eyes as she has done before. By staying put, Sally realises some important things:

- First, no-one seems that bothered. No-one looks at her or says anything critical about her not controlling her child.
- Second, Jack quickly settles down and eventually goes to sleep in his pram. In fact at the checkout another mother says to her how peaceful he looks.

Finally, make a summary of all the information you have about the upsetting thought.

Summary

In this workbook you have learned to:

- Notice patterns of extreme and unhelpful thinking that worsen how you feel.

- Change this kind of thinking so it's less upsetting.

The approach you have worked through will work for any unhelpful thoughts that make you feel worse. By labelling, stepping back from and challenging these thoughts, you will begin to change the way you see yourself, the way things are right now and in the future.

Q What have I learnt from this workbook?

Q What do I want to try *next*?

Putting into practice what you have learned

You will find blank thought practice worksheets at the end of this workbook. Please copy them if you need more. You can also download more sheets for free from the Five Areas website (**www.fiveareas.com**).

Getting the most from the thought worksheets

To get the most from the worksheets:

- Practise using the approach whenever you notice your mood is changing unhelpfully. In this way, you'll find it easier to notice and change your extreme and unhelpful thinking.

- Try to notice and challenge your unhelpful thoughts **as soon as possible** after you notice your mood change.

- If you can't do this immediately, try to think yourself back into the situation so that you are as clear as possible in your answers later on when you do this task.

- With practice you'll find that you can work out what are the most helpful parts of this workbook for you and use them to help you in everyday life.

My notes

Practice sheet

My Five Areas thought review of a time when I felt worse

Please write in your thoughts in all Five Areas.

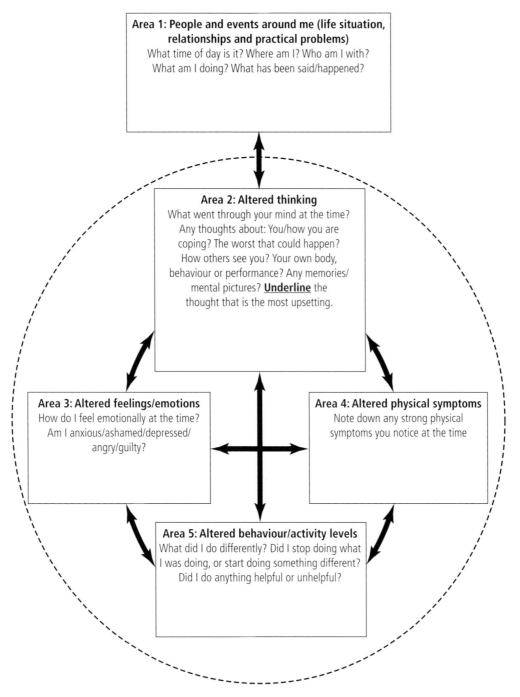

Area 1: People and events around me (life situation, relationships and practical problems)
What time of day is it? Where am I? Who am I with?
What am I doing? What has been said/happened?

Area 2: Altered thinking
What went through your mind at the time?
Any thoughts about: You/how you are
coping? The worst that could happen?
How others see you? Your own body,
behaviour or performance? Any memories/
mental pictures? **Underline** the
thought that is the most upsetting.

Area 3: Altered feelings/emotions
How do I feel emotionally at the time?
Am I anxious/ashamed/depressed/
angry/guilty?

Area 4: Altered physical symptoms
Note down any strong physical
symptoms you notice at the time

Area 5: Altered behaviour/activity levels
What did I do differently? Did I stop doing what
I was doing, or start doing something different?
Did I do anything helpful or unhelpful?

Summary: The key steps of the thought review

Use the responses below that work for you.

1. **Label the thought** as 'just one of those unhelpful thoughts'.

- Am I being my own worst critic? (Bias against yourself)
- Am I focusing on the bad in situations? (A negative mental filter)
- Am I making negative predictions about the future? (A gloomy view of the future)
- Am I jumping to the very worst conclusion? (Catastrophising)
- Am I second-guessing that others see me badly without checking if it's actually true? (Mind-reading)
- Am I **taking unfair responsibility** for things that aren't really my fault/taking all the blame?
- Am I using unhelpful **must/should/ought/got to** statements? (Making extreme statements or setting impossible standards).

2. **Stop, think and reflect**: Don't get caught up in the thought.

3. **Move on**:

- Don't be put off from what you were going to do.
- Keep active. Face your fears.
- Keep to your plan. Respond helpfully.
- Don't be bullied. Act against the upsetting thought and see what happens.

4. Respond by giving yourself a **truly caring response** – for example what would someone who loved you wholly and totally say?

5. Question the thought by asking yourself the seven thought challenge questions:

- What would I tell a friend who said the same thing?

- Am I basing this on how I feel rather than the facts?

- What would other people say?

- Am I looking at the whole picture?

- Does it really matter so much?

- What would I say about this looking back six months from the future?

- Do I apply one set of standards to myself and another to others?

Finally, make a summary of everything you have learned.

Remember: This process takes time and practise to build your confidence in using the approach.

 A downloadable credit-card sized version of this summary is available free of charge from the Five Areas website (**www.fiveareas.com**).

Overcoming Postnatal Depression

A Five Areas Approach

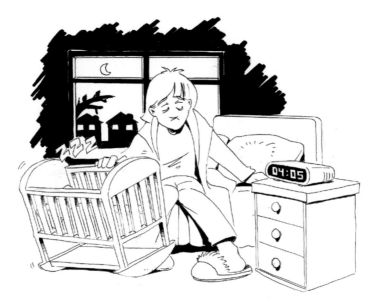

Overcoming sleep problems

www.livinglifetothefull.com
www.fiveareas.com

Dr Chris Williams, Dr Roch Cantwell and Karen Robertson

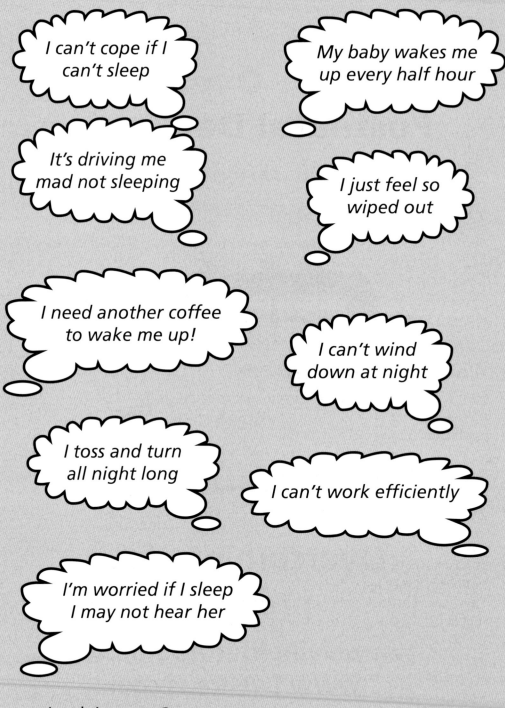

… is this you?

If so … this workbook is for you.

In this workbook you will:

- Learn about sleep and sleeplessness.

- Learn about some common causes of sleep problems.

- Learn how to record your sleep pattern and identify things that worsen your sleep.

- Learn about making some changes that will help you sleep better.

What is enough sleep?

How much sleep you need depends on the person. Some people function well after sleeping only four to six hours a day whereas others need as many as 10 or 12 hours a day. Both extremes are quite normal.

Sleep problems are common and affect lots of people.

What causes sleeplessness?

Most people have problems sleeping from time to time. Sleep problems often start after an upsetting life event, or they can be a result of your lifestyle. Many psychological problems can also upset sleep. These include anxiety, depression, anger, guilt, shame and stress. Stress can be caused by, for example, problems in relationships. Some people who have depression find that it takes them several hours to fall asleep. They may also wake up several hours earlier than normal, feeling as if they haven't rested at all or feeling on edge.

Having a baby, and also having postnatal depression are two common causes of sleeplessness among mothers. First, your baby won't have a sleep routine to start with. It may take them several months or even longer to sleep through the night. Second, feeding during the night disrupts your sleep pattern until your baby is old enough to eat or drink enough to see them through the night.

Speak to your health visitor for advice on healthy sleep routines for you and your baby. A widely recommended book that you may find helpful to establish a regular sleeping pattern for your baby – and help teach them ways of settling and soothing themselves – is *The Secrets of the Baby Whisperer: How to Calm, Connect and Communicate with Your Baby* by Tracy Hogg.

A Five Areas assessment of sleeplessness

Many things can affect your sleep and so also affect your life. This section describes the things that can affect each of the five areas of your life.

Area 1: People and events around you

Your baby and your bed

Experts recommend that you should make your baby sleep in the same room as you at night during the first few months of life. The Scottish Cot Death Trust (**www.sidscotland.org.uk**) also makes the following recommendations to reduce the risks of cot death:

- Place baby on the back to sleep.
- Do not let anyone smoke in the same room as your baby.
- Avoid overheating baby.
- Keep baby's head uncovered – place baby's feet at the bottom of the cot.
- Do not share a bed with your baby if you have been drinking alcohol, take drugs or if you are a smoker.

Problems with noise

Some noises, such as your baby's crying, can only be changed slowly over time. You may, however, be able to tackle other sources of noise. For example if you have noisy neighbours, could you or someone else ask them to turn down their television or music? Have you thought about fitting double glazing or plastic sheeting inside windows to reduce noise? This needn't be expensive and many reasonably priced options are available.

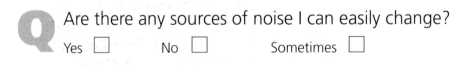

Q Are there any sources of noise I can easily change?

Yes ☐   No ☐   Sometimes ☐

Your physical environment

- Is your bed comfortable?
- What about the temperature of the room where you sleep? If the room is either very cold or very hot this might make it hard to go to sleep.
- Is there too much light in the room? If bright lights such as streetlights come through your curtains, this can also prevent you sleeping.

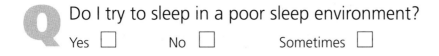

Q Do I try to sleep in a poor sleep environment?

Yes ☐ No ☐ Sometimes ☐

If you answered 'Yes' or 'Sometimes', you could try looking at some of these things to help you sleep better.

Poor mattress

If your mattress is quite old, can you turn it over, rotate it or perhaps even change it. You may be able to add extra support, such as a board or old door underneath it.

Too hot/cold

If your bedroom is too hot, try opening a window or using a fan. If it's too cold, think about using an extra blanket or duvet. Or you could think about insulation, draught excluders, secondary or double glazing.

Problems with excessive light

Consider the thickness of your curtains. Have you thought about adding a thicker lining or blackout lining? If this may not be possible, for example because of the cost involved, a black plastic bin bag can work well as a blackout blind. It can be stapled or stuck to the curtain rail or window surround. If you use sticky Velcro, you can easily put this up at night and take it down during the day.

Area 2: Altered thinking

Anxious thoughts are a common cause of sleeplessness. You may have anxious thoughts about your baby or life in general. For example:

- You may worry about not sleeping or not hearing your baby during the night.
- You may worry that your baby will become ill or stop breathing.
- You may worry that you will not be able to sleep at all – or that sleeplessness will reduce your ability to concentrate the next day.
- Your fears get blown out of proportion and prevent you going off to sleep.
- Another common fear is that your brain or your body will be harmed by lack of sleep.

Usually as you try to go off to sleep, your tension levels go down, so your body and brain begin to relax and drop off to sleep. In contrast, when you're anxious, your brain becomes overly alert. You end up mulling over things again and again. This is the exact opposite of what's needed to go to sleep. Worrying thoughts are therefore both a cause and effect of poor sleep.

Q Do I worry about things in general?

Yes ☐   No ☐   Sometimes ☐

📌 Task

If you answered 'Yes', read the *Noticing and changing extreme and unhelpful thinking* workbook.

Q Do I worry about not sleeping?

Yes ☐   No ☐   Sometimes ☐

If you answered 'Yes' or 'Sometimes', write down your worries on a notepad. You will need to challenge any fears that are out of proportion about the impact of not sleeping. It's helpful to know that research shows that most people don't need very much sleep at all to be physically and mentally healthy. When people who may have poor sleep are asked to try to sleep in a sleep research laboratory, they may actually sleep far more than they think. Sometimes people who are in a light level of sleep dream that they are awake. So you may be sleeping more than you think.

It's helpful to know that not sleeping enough doesn't have a very big effect on your brain or your body. It is possible to function well with very little sleep each night.

Q Do I have extreme fears about the impact of not sleeping?

Yes ☐   No ☐   Sometimes ☐

Extreme (catastrophic) fears can themselves cause increased wakefulness, and actually prevent you going off to sleep. It is important for you to know that these thoughts are extreme, inaccurate and unhelpful. Although you might feel tired and irritable, this doesn't necessarily affect your ability to do things around the house or at work.

Task

If worrying thoughts are a problem for you, read the *Noticing and changing extreme and unhelpful thinking* workbook.

Area 3: Altered physical problems

Pain, itching or other physical symptoms can cause sleeplessness. Tackling these physical symptoms will help with your sleep problems.

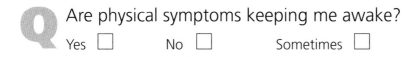 Are physical symptoms keeping me awake?

Yes ☐   No ☐   Sometimes ☐

If you answered 'Yes' or 'Sometimes', please see your doctor as you may need medical treatment for your symptoms. Sometimes if you have depression or anxiety, your physical symptoms can feel worse. Your doctor then may offer you treatment for your low or anxious mood to help reduce the physical symptoms.

Area 4: Altered feelings

Many feelings can be linked to sleeplessness.

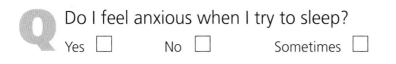 Do I feel anxious when I try to sleep?

Yes ☐   No ☐   Sometimes ☐

If you answered 'Yes' or 'Sometimes', remember that anxiety is a common cause of sleeplessness. It often triggers your body's fear response causing adrenaline to flow. Adrenaline is a substance produced by your body that makes you feel fidgety or restless. You may notice physical symptoms such as your heartbeat and breathing getting faster, a churning feeling in your stomach or tension throughout your body. Your anxiety therefore acts to keep you alert. This is the opposite of what you want when you're trying to fall asleep. Sometimes you may become anxious about sleeping (for example if you have nightmares or wake up feeling panicky). Find out more about dealing with anxiety in the *Anxiety and avoidance* workbook and at **www.livinglifetothefull.com**.

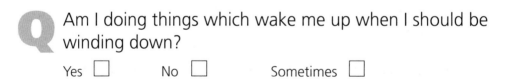

Am I feeling depressed, upset or low in mood and do I no longer enjoy things as before?

Yes ☐   No ☐   Sometimes ☐

If you answered 'Yes' or 'Sometimes', remember that depression is a common cause of sleeplessness. For example, when you are feeling depressed you may find that it takes you several hours to get to sleep. You may wake up several hours earlier than normal feeling unrested or on edge. Having treatment for your depression can often be helpful for improving your sleep.

Other emotions such as shame, guilt and anger can also cause sleeplessness.

Area 5: Altered behaviour: unhelpful behaviours

Preparing for sleep

The time leading up to sleep is very important. Try to build in a '**wind-down**' time in the evening when you are less active and engaged in less stimulating activity. Physical over-activity such as exercising, eating too much, using the computer or watching TV just before going to bed can keep you awake. Sometimes people watch TV while lying in bed. This may help them wind down, but many people become more alert and so it adds to their sleep problems.

Am I doing things which wake me up when I should be winding down?

Yes ☐   No ☐   Sometimes ☐

If you answered 'Yes' or 'Sometimes', keep your bed as a place for sleep. Don't lie on your bed watching TV, working or worrying. This will only wake you up and prevent you sleeping. You'll also need to decide whether listening to a radio or music helps you go to sleep.

What about caffeine?

Caffeine is a chemical found in cola drinks, coffee, tea, some hot chocolate and some herbal drinks. It causes you to be more alert. People who have lots of caffeine for several weeks can get addicted to it. It also reduces your sleep quality. There is a real risk that you can get into a vicious circle, in which tiredness causes you to drink more caffeine to keep alert. Then the caffeine itself affects your sleep and worsens the original tiredness. Try not to drink more than five cups of strong coffee or equivalent a day

Key point

It is important to know that caffeine stays in your body for a few hours before it is broken down by your body or it leaves in your urine. This means that you should avoid drinking caffeine drinks in the few hours leading up to bed.

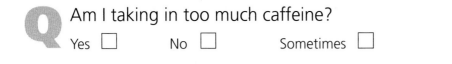

Am I taking in too much caffeine?

Yes ☐   No ☐   Sometimes ☐

If you answered 'Yes' or 'Sometimes', you should reduce the amount of caffeine-containing drinks you take. Do this in a step-by-step way, for example by switching slowly to decaffeinated cola, coffees or teas. Definitely don't have caffeine before sleep. Both caffeine and nicotine (the chemical in cigarettes) will keep you awake. Some people find that a warm, milky drink can help them fall asleep.

What about alcohol?

Sometimes people drink alcohol to reduce their feelings of tension and to help them get off to sleep. But this can actually cause problems such as anxiety, depression and sleeplessness. Also, drinking too much may cause you to go to the toilet more than usual at night. This will also keep you awake. You can find out more about the impact of alcohol and street drugs in the workbook *Alcohol, drugs and your baby*.

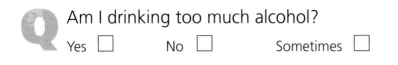

Am I drinking too much alcohol?

Yes ☐   No ☐   Sometimes ☐

If you answered 'Yes' or 'Sometimes', you can avoid getting up in the night to use the toilet by reducing the amount you drink before going to bed. If you drink above the healthy drink range (see the workbook *Alcohol, drugs and your baby*), try to cut down in a slow step-by-step manner. Discuss how best to do this with your GP or healthcare worker.

What about your sleep pattern?

If you aren't sleeping well, you can be tempted to go to bed either much earlier or much later than normal.

Usually when people have sleep problems, they are advised to cut down on napping. This is because napping is another habit that can end up backfiring by upsetting your natural sleep–wake cycle. But if your baby wakes up often during the night and sleeps during the day then it's understandable to take some sleep when you can. When your baby starts to settle into a more regular sleep–wake cycle, it is a good time for you to cut down on your own daytime sleeps.

A regular sleep pattern can help to maintain a clear start and end to the day. Try therefore to get up before 9 a.m. and to sleep before about 11 p.m.

Q Do I have a disrupted sleep pattern (no regular time to bed/getting up)?

Yes ☐   No ☐   Sometimes ☐

If you answered 'Yes' or 'Sometimes', set yourself regular sleep times. Get up at a set time even if you have slept poorly. Try to teach your body what time to fall asleep and what time to get up. Go to sleep some time between 10 p.m. and midnight. Try to get up at a sensible time between 6 a.m. and 9 a.m. Adjust these times to fit your own circumstances and your baby's sleep pattern.

Tossing and turning in bed and clock watching

Q Do you find yourself lying awake in bed tossing and turning, waking your partner up to talk ('Are you awake? ...'), or just watching the clock?

Yes ☐   No ☐   Sometimes ☐

If you answered 'Yes' or 'Sometimes', then some practical changes can help, such as moving the clock so you can't see it. It can still be in the room so that you can set an alarm or reach it if you have to. Some mothers find they constantly get up to check their baby monitor for breathing, or the room temperature on the readout (if your monitor shows this). Again, try to have an appropriate balance. If your baby is ill, cold, too hot or distressed then you will need to get up to check them. However it's important to build confidence and not get up when all that you can hear is simply heavy breathing or occasional coughs.

Recording your sleep

🖈 **Task**

You may find it helpful to use a **Sleep diary** for a few days this week as you use this workbook. A blank sleep diary is included at the end of this workbook. You can copy out the headings or photocopy the diary. By completing the diary you will be able to identify what important factors affect your sleep.

Carrying out your own Five Areas assessment

Look at the Five Areas assessment in the figure on the next page. Write in all the things you have identified that affect your sleep. These are possible targets for change.

Five Areas assessment of factors affecting my sleep

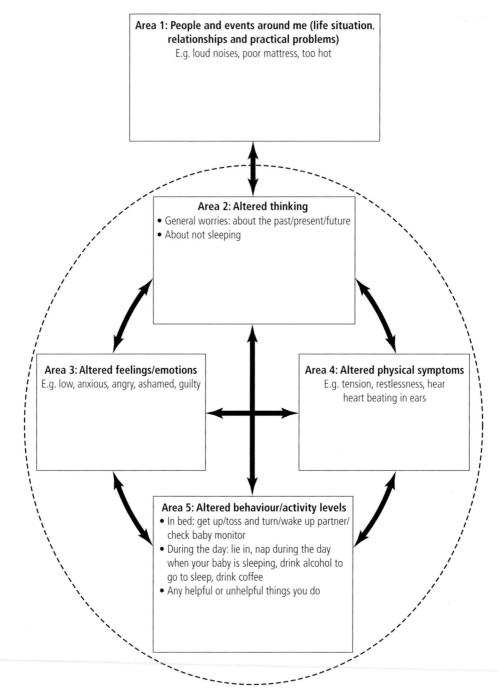

Area 1: People and events around me (life situation, relationships and practical problems)
E.g. loud noises, poor mattress, too hot

Area 2: Altered thinking
• General worries: about the past/present/future
• About not sleeping

Area 3: Altered feelings/emotions
E.g. low, anxious, angry, ashamed, guilty

Area 4: Altered physical symptoms
E.g. tension, restlessness, hear heart beating in ears

Area 5: Altered behaviour/activity levels
• In bed: get up/toss and turn/wake up partner/ check baby monitor
• During the day: lie in, nap during the day when your baby is sleeping, drink alcohol to go to sleep, drink coffee
• Any helpful or unhelpful things you do

Overcoming sleeplessness

Use the checklists below to find out about things you can do to get rid of your sleep problems.

Sleep checklist: Some things to do and not do

Some things to do in the run-up to bed and during the day	Tick here if this affects your life – even if just sometimes	Some changes you can make and resources you can use
Plan a wind-down time each evening	☐	See earlier in this workbook: warm bran-based milky drinks may help. Think about having a bath and listening to relaxing music. If you like candles or scented oils try using those
Have a regular time to go to bed and to get up	☐	See earlier in this workbook (page 320)
Tackle the things that you know affect your sleep environment (for example external noise, mattress)	☐	See earlier in this workbook. If your neighbours cause the noise, the *Practical problem solving* and *Being assertive* workbooks will help you find ways of dealing with this problem. Also think about your surroundings (noise, light levels, temperature, and also the comfort of your bed). Plan changes to your room/mattress as needed
Reduce your general life pressures	☐	Say no – balance demands you put on yourself. Allow space and time for yourself. The *Being assertive* workbook may help you with this
Stop, think and reflect on worrying thoughts about the past, the present and the future, and also about sleep	☐	If worrying thoughts keep you awake, write the worries down. Decide to worry or think them through tomorrow during the day (see note at the end of the table). Use the *Noticing and changing extreme and unhelpful thinking* workbook to put your thoughts into perspective the next day

Some things to do in the run-up to bed and during the day	Tick here if this affects your life – even if just sometimes	Some changes you can make and resources you can use
Live reasonably healthily. People who are fitter generally sleep better	☐	It might sound strange to say this, but over-doing healthy living may become unhealthy, for example doing too much exercise before sleeping. Try to live healthily but not obsessively so
Use relaxation tapes or techniques if you find them helpful	☐	You may wish to try the free downloadable relaxation resources using Anxiety Control Training (originally developed by Dr Philip Snaith). See our support website for this book (**www.fiveareas.com**)

Some things *not* to do in the run-up to bed and during the day	Tick here if this affects your life – even if just sometimes	Some changes you can make and resources you can use
Drinking too much alcohol or caffeine (or smoking) just before bed	☐	Alcohol causes sleep to be shallow and unrefreshing. It can also make you wake up more to use the toilet. Don't drink too many cola drinks, or too much coffee, tea or hot chocolate, which contain caffeine. Switch to decaffeinated drinks or water. Nicotine in cigarettes causes sleeplessness too. Don't smoke just before bed
Doing things that stimulate you mentally or physically in the run-up to sleep (for example using the computer, or watching an exciting film)	☐	You can of course do all these things, but stop doing them at least an hour before going to bed. Avoid doing them in bed too

Some things *not* to do in the run-up to bed and during the day	Tick here if this affects your life – even if just sometimes	Some changes you can make and resources you can use
Let problems build up so that you worry about them at night	☐	Write down your problems to deal with tomorrow. This approach was originally developed by Dr Tom Borkevic, who advises that you write a diary list of worries. Write them down and then plan a specific *'worry time'* the following day. Many people find that the worries become a lot smaller in the light of day
Respond in ways that end up backfiring or worsening things (for example lying in during the day, napping beyond the time it's helpful)	☐	Try to re-set your body clock by getting up at a set time each day. It's understandable that you would like to take naps when you can early on after your baby is born. But it's important to avoid napping and to go to bed at roughly the same time each day once they get into a more regular routine
Don't look for answers to sleeplessness in sleeping tablets	☐	These tablets are not advisable long term

Don't expect to change everything immediately. But with practice, you can make helpful changes to your sleep pattern. If you find it hard at first, just do what you can.

Your own Five Areas assessment may have helped you identify the problems you have at present and the table above will have provided you with hints and tips in each of your main problem areas.

Summary

In this workbook you have learnt about:

- Sleep and sleeplessness.

- Some common causes of sleep problems.

- How to record your sleep pattern and identify things that worsen your sleep.

- Making some changes that will help you sleep better.

Q What have I learnt from this?

Q What do I want to try *next*?

Putting what you have learned into practice

Look back at the **sleep checklist of things to do and not do** on pages 323–325. Plan to make changes in how you prepare for sleep and what you do once you are in bed.

Write down what you're going to do this week, to put into practice what you have learnt.

My practice plan

 What changes am I going to make?

 When am I going to do it?

Q What problems could arise, and how can I sort these?

Apply the **Questions for effective change** to your plan.

Q Is my planned task one that:

- Will be useful for understanding or changing how I am?

    Yes ☐   No ☐

- Is a specific task so that I will know when I have done it?

    Yes ☐   No ☐

- Is realistic, practical and achievable?

    Yes ☐   No ☐

- Makes clear what I am going to do and when I am going to do it.

  Yes ☐   No ☐

- Is an activity that won't be easily blocked or prevented by practical problems?

  Yes ☐   No ☐

- Will help me to learn useful things even if it doesn't work out perfectly?

  Yes ☐   No ☐

Remember to review your progress in making these changes weekly, and to make sure the changes are practical and achievable.

My notes

My sleep diary

Time when you are in bed and trying to sleep	Record when you are **asleep** with an 'X'	Record when your baby is **asleep** with an 'X'	**When in bed**, record any **thoughts/images** that go through your mind and keep you awake (for example worries, fears about sleeping or the impact of not sleeping)	Record any **activities** you do that relate to sleep **Before bed**: alcohol, caffeine, smoking, exercise, daytime napping, computer games, watching scary films, sleeping in **In bed**: reading, listening to the radio, disturbing other people, tossing/turning, getting up and going downstairs, etc.
8.00 p.m.–9.59 p.m.				
10.00 p.m.–11.59 p.m.				
12.00 a.m.–1.59 a.m.				
2.00 a.m.–3.59 a.m.				
4.00 a.m.–5.59 a.m.				
6.00 a.m.–7.59 a.m.				
8.00 a.m.–9.59 a.m.				
10.00 a.m.–11.59 a.m.				
12.00 p.m.–1.59 p.m.				
2.00 p.m.–3.59 p.m.				
4.00 p.m.–5.59 p.m.				
6.00 p.m.–7.59 p.m.				

Overcoming Postnatal Depression
A Five Areas Approach

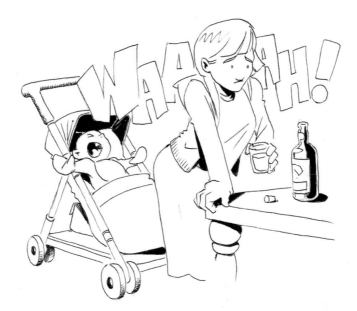

Alcohol, drugs and your baby

www.livinglifetothefull.com
www.fiveareas.com

Dr Chris Williams, Dr Roch Cantwell and
Karen Robertson

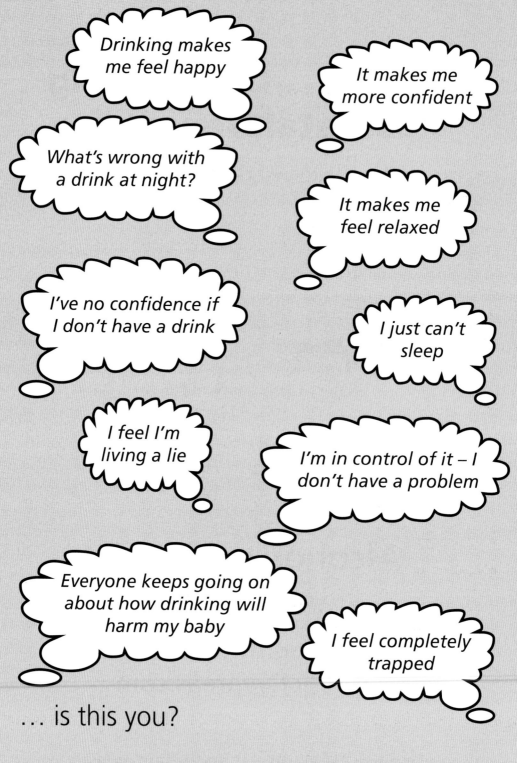

… is this you?

If so … this workbook is for you.

If you are misusing alcohol or street drugs you have a serious problem. And it can cause a serious problem for your baby too.

In this workbook you will:

- Learn some useful facts about alcohol and street drugs.

- Discover how alcohol and street drugs can affect you and your family.

- Work out what effect they're having on you.

- Plan some next steps to bring about change if you have a problem.

Alcohol and street drugs are widely used socially – for fun, for relaxation and for enjoyment. But they can both be misused. Also, buying street drugs is illegal.

Using alcohol

Surveys show that many people have drink problems. Having a baby can sometimes be a time when people decide they want a fresh start – and manage to cut back. But sometimes it can be hard drinking less. Have you been drinking to fit in with the crowd, enjoy the effects of drink, or to block out uncomfortable feelings? If you've been drinking a lot of alcohol for weeks or months it can be affecting your mood, your body and your relationships. It can also affect your baby.

The recommended **highest levels of alcohol for adults** to drink in one week:

- 22 units for women

- 28 units for men.

The amounts are less (and sometimes much less) for younger people depending on your age and weight.

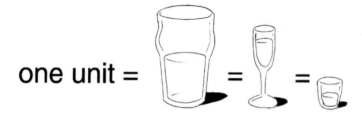

one unit =

1 unit is = half a pint of bitter or lager, or 1 small glass of wine, or one measure of spirits (for example, whisky or gin).

Key point

These values vary because stronger lagers or beers, or fortified wines, contain far more than one unit of alcohol. So always look at the back of the bottle where you'll find how many units of alcohol there are in standard size glasses for that particular drink.

Using street drugs

People use street drugs for similar reasons to alcohol. There are lots of different street drugs. And even when you think you may be buying one type on the street, it may be contaminated with all sorts of other drugs.

The effects of different drugs vary, but there are some effects which are common to all drugs and alcohol.

 For more information about street drugs, visit the Talk to Frank website (**www.talktofrank.com**).

Recording what you drink and what drugs you use

 Task

Everybody is different. Whether you are drinking or taking street drugs, a **good first step** is to record how much you use. Remember that most people tend to think they have a lot less than they really have.

Q How many units of alcohol do you drink?

In one day:

- What drink? _____

- How much? _____

- How many times? _____

In one week?

- What drink? _____

- How much? _____

- How many times? _____

How many units is that per week? _____ units

How much are you spending a week on drinks? £_____

Q What street drugs are you taking?

In one day:

- What drug? _____

- How much? _____

- How many times? _____

In one week?

- What drug? _____

- How much? _____

- How many times? _____

How much are you spending per week on drugs? £_____

The best way of finding out how much you drink or use in a week is to keep a **diary**. You'll find one at the back of this workbook (page 347). Try to **record each and every time** you drink alcohol or use drugs. At the end of the week, add up the amount you have taken.

How alcohol and drugs affect your baby

While your baby is growing during your pregnancy

Both alcohol and drugs can affect your baby's weight and growth, and also may affect the development of their brain and body. If your baby has become used to high levels of alcohol or drugs in your body during pregnancy, they may be unwell when they are born and require special care supports.

After your baby is born

If you continue to drink a lot after your baby is born, your baby is affected in two main ways:

● First by the effect on you. Drink may make you more prone to accidents, clumsiness or unwise decisions. You may not be able to meet your baby's needs when you have been drinking. Your baby may come to harm as a result.

● If you are breastfeeding, breast milk can contain alcohol or drugs. This can affect your baby's alertness, ability to learn and their development.

It's important to tell your doctor or your midwife if you have been misusing alcohol or drugs.

How alcohol and drugs affect you

When you drink a large amount of alcohol or take a large dose of drugs – or regularly drink or take drugs at low doses – you can have several problems. Some of these are described below.

Thinking/psychological changes

People often drink or use drugs to improve how they feel. But actually these things can cause you to have a low mood and prevent your postnatal depression getting better.

Drinking and taking drugs can:

- Worsen worry and panic attacks.

- Lead to sudden bouts of confusion or violence.

- Damage your concentration and memory so that you find it hard to learn and remember new information.

- Worsen your ability to fall asleep and to have a refreshing night's sleep.

- Cause you to become fearful, and increasingly suspicious and mistrustful of others.

- Lead to addiction with craving if you stop taking them abruptly.

Drinking and taking drugs can also make you feel irritable. Your personality changes, but in such a subtle way that you don't realise that you're changing as a result of your habit. You may also become withdrawn, and stop taking interest in your baby, other people or the things around you. You could even become suspicious of everything around you.

People can occasionally develop severe psychiatric (mental health) disorders that can become long term, such as having hallucinations (seeing or hearing things that aren't there) or delusions (believing something is true when it clearly isn't). These illnesses can be terrifying to have. They also pose a high risk not only to your safety but also to the safety of others you feel strongly about.

 Do you have any of the mental health symptoms described above?

(You may need to ask people around you.)

Yes ☐   No ☐   Sometimes ☐

Physical changes

- The most common symptom of drinking too much is having a hangover. This includes feeling sick, having headaches and becoming dehydrated (this is when your body doesn't have the fluids it needs to function properly).

- Both alcohol and drugs can lead to addiction. If then you suddenly stop either, you get **withdrawal symptoms** such as sweatiness and feeling sick. If you take a lot of alcohol or drugs, you can become dependent on them (alcohol/drug dependency). You can also become dependent on the so-called 'soft' drugs, for example cannabis – some types of which are not 'soft' in effect at all.

- If someone drinks or uses drugs at a high level for some time and then suddenly stops them, there is a high risk of serious withdrawal. This is a serious medical condition. Symptoms of withdrawal include confusion, agitation and hallucinations. The person may even go into a coma, or have fits or wet themselves.

- Alcohol can cause damage to parts of your body. For example it can cause stomach ulcers (holes in the lining of your stomach) and it can damage your liver. It can also damage your brain so that you start having epileptic fits. Other important body organs such as the pancreas can also be damaged, causing you pain.

- Drugs can cause **lung cancer** and heart problems, or you can have a stroke. You can also start having fits or your body temperature regulation can get upset. They can also cause you to get suddenly confused. People can even die all of a sudden as drugs can be toxic to many body organs.

- Taking drugs can reduce your ability to fight off infections or serious disease.

Q Do you have any of the physical symptoms described above?

Yes ☐   No ☐   Sometimes ☐

Social changes

- You may have problems at home such as **arguments** with family and friends.

- You may get into **debt**.

- You may struggle even more to look after your baby. Money you should be spending on food, nappies and clothes may be spent instead on drink or drugs. You may neglect your baby as a result. This could lead to social services becoming involved to offer assessment and support if they are concerned about how you are caring for your baby.

- **Accidents and violence** are also common social consequences of alcohol dependency.

Q Do you have any of the social symptoms described above?

Yes ☐   No ☐   Sometimes ☐

Based on your answers to all the questions above:

Q Overall, do you think that you're having drink/drug problems?

Yes ☐   No ☐   Sometimes ☐

Key point

If you have answered 'Yes' or 'Sometimes' to this question then this is an alert that you need to make some changes. **Drinking or using drugs in ways that can harm you or your baby** is likely to cause you increasing problems in each of the areas described above. **You need to tackle your problem now**. Don't be tempted to downplay or ignore things and believe it isn't a problem. **Ignoring things is often part of the problem.**

Example: Julia's drinking

Julia has started to drink more to try to cope with symptoms such as low mood and tension about things. Her drinking is now affecting both her and her baby Ben.

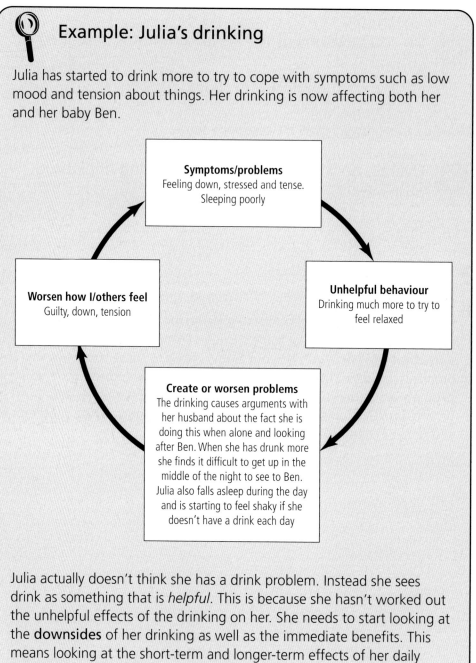

Symptoms/problems
Feeling down, stressed and tense.
Sleeping poorly

Unhelpful behaviour
Drinking much more to try to feel relaxed

Create or worsen problems
The drinking causes arguments with her husband about the fact she is doing this when alone and looking after Ben. When she has drunk more she finds it difficult to get up in the middle of the night to see to Ben. Julia also falls asleep during the day and is starting to feel shaky if she doesn't have a drink each day

Worsen how I/others feel
Guilty, down, tension

Julia actually doesn't think she has a drink problem. Instead she sees drink as something that is *helpful*. This is because she hasn't worked out the unhelpful effects of the drinking on her. She needs to start looking at the **downsides** of her drinking as well as the immediate benefits. This means looking at the short-term and longer-term effects of her daily drinking on herself, Ben and her partner Dave.

How your drinking affects you

> ## Example: How is Julia's drinking affecting her?
>
> In the short term:
>
> - **Physically**: Julia is noticing she feels shaky if she doesn't have a drink every day.
> - **Psychologically**: She feels it makes her more relaxed and helps her sleep at night to begin with. But then she wakes up and has to go to the toilet. So she feels too tired to get up in the morning and look after Ben. She also feels more depressed in the morning when she's been drinking more the night before.
> - **Socially**: Julia's partner Dave is worried about her, and they keep having arguments about her drinking. She worries it's affecting how she looks after Ben.

Key point

Both *helpful* and *unhelpful* behaviours make us feel better in the short term. But in the longer term, our unhelpful behaviours – such as heavy drinking – backfire. They worsen how we or others feel. They become part of our problem. The good news is that if this applies to you, you can make changes.

 Task

Now think about your own drinking or drug use or both.

Q How does my drinking or drug use affect me and the people around me in the short term and longer term?

Short term

- Physically:

- Psychologically:

- Socially (on you and others including your baby):

Longer term (look back to over the past six to 12 months)

- Physically:

- Psychologically:

- Socially (on you and others):

If after reading this workbook you have discovered that your drinking or drug use is causing harm to you or others, then **you need to tackle it**.

 What have I learnt from this workbook?

 What do I want to try *next*?

How to make changes

Try to reduce your overall intake of alcohol or drugs each week. Do this slowly in steady steps over several weeks. If possible, plan to eventually have **at least two days** each week without any drink or drugs to allow your body to recover. Discuss your goals and how to achieve this with your doctor.

If you're drinking or using street drugs at a far higher level

If you stop drinking or taking the drugs too quickly, you may notice some symptoms of withdrawal. This is probably the reason why so many people don't manage to tackle this problem. But it's possible to make changes – and it's even more important to do so if you're having a lot of drink or drugs.

To change yourself successfully you need to cut down the amount you're taking in a **slow, step-by-step manner**. You may find the *Unhelpful things you do* workbook helpful for some ideas of how to plan this, so that it happens. But if you're taking drugs or drinking alcohol at higher levels, it's best to make these changes together with some closer help and advice from your GP, health visitor, your local drug or alcohol support services or other healthcare practitioner.

Key point

If you regularly use street drugs, or drink a lot of alcohol, please can you discuss this with someone who can help.

Extra resources

Look at your local *Yellow Pages*, and also the following national organisations:

1. **NHS Direct (England and Wales)**. NHS Direct will help and advise on any aspect of drug and alcohol use (tel: 0845 46 47; **www.nhsdirect.nhs.uk**).

2. **NHS24 (Scotland)**. If you live in Scotland ring NHS24 for advice and assessment (tel: 0845 424 242; **www.nhs24.com**).

3. **Royal College of Psychiatrists**. The College has an information sheet about drugs and alcohol (**www.rcpsych.ac.uk**).

4. **Talk to Frank**. This website has stories, information and resources about drugs. It also has information for family and friends. You can talk on the phone and ask for information from a counsellor or you can email or access help online (tel: 0800 776 600; **www.talktofrank.com**). Please note that Frank is not a real person but the website is a way for you to get advice and information about drugs.

5. **Alcohol Focus Scotland (www.alcohol-focus-scotland.org.uk)** and **Drinks Aware (www.drinkaware.co.uk)** are two other useful websites.

Summary

In this workbook you have learnt:

- Some useful facts about alcohol and street drugs.

- How alcohol and street drugs can affect you and your family.

- How you can work out what effects they're having on you.

- How to plan some next steps to bring about change if you have a problem.

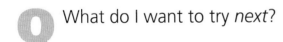 What have I learnt from this workbook?

What do I want to try *next*?

My notes

Drink/street drug diary: my week

Day and date	Morning	Afternoon	Evening	Total units or cost
Monday				Total units/amount per day = Cost/day £ =
Tuesday				Total units/amount per day = Cost/day £ =
Wednesday				Total units/amount per day = Cost/day £ =
Thursday				Total units/amount per day = Cost/day £ =
Friday				Total units/amount per day = Cost/day £ =
Saturday				Total units/amount per day = Cost/day £ =
Sunday				Total units/amount per day = Cost/day £ =
Weekly total				**Units = Cost =**

Key point

Remember to record everything you drink/take. If you are drinking/using drugs on a regular basis and/or at a high dose, it may prevent you getting better.

Overcoming Postnatal Depression
A Five Areas Approach

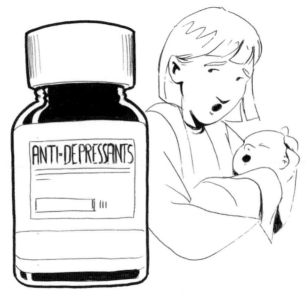

Understanding and using anti-depressant medication

www.livinglifetothefull.com
www.fiveareas.com

Dr Chris Williams, Dr Roch Cantwell and
Karen Robertson

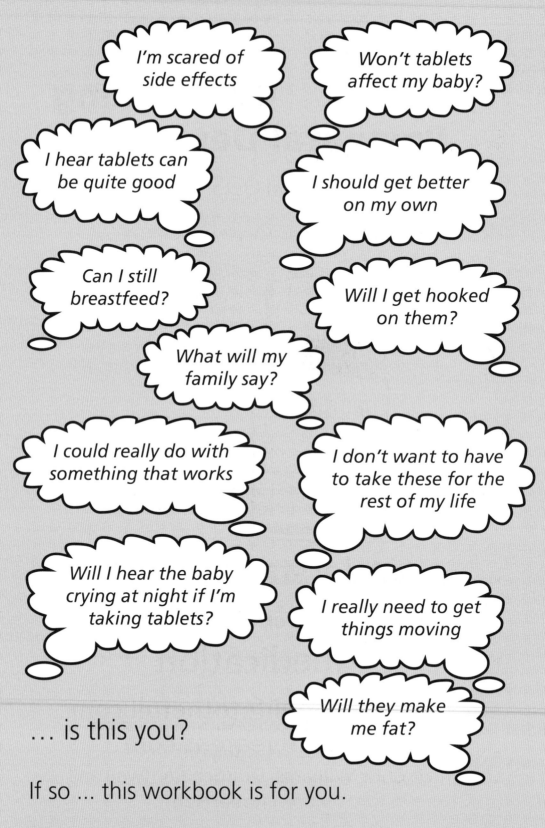

... is this you?

If so ... this workbook is for you.

In this workbook you will:

- Find out about how anti-depressants are used for postnatal depression.

- Get the answers to some common questions about anti-depressants.

- Get some useful hints and tips to get the best out of your medication.

- Learn how to think through the pros and cons of medication, if this is being suggested for you.

How do tablets fit in with your treatment?

National guidelines in the UK recommend that people with depression should be offered treatments other than medication (for example, psychological or 'talking' treatments) at first. But anti-depressant medications can be helpful as part of a **package of care** (that is, provided you're also having other treatments at the same time).

Your doctor can tell you more about the different types of anti-depressants available.

Key point

If you're already using an anti-depressant you shouldn't stop them if they are helping. You should continue to take them as originally planned, and all your treatment decisions will still be made with your doctor.

When are tablets helpful?

Anti-depressants are helpful if you have moderate or severe symptoms of depression. These include:

- Feeling low or noticing you no longer enjoy things most of the time, for at least two weeks.

- Several of the physical changes of depression (for example: low energy, reduced concentration, changes in your sleep pattern or appetite).

- Feeling very agitated, suspicious or panicking a lot.

- Getting suicidal ideas, that is, where you can't see a future.

When are tablets not helpful?

Usually anti-depressants aren't helpful for problems of mildly low mood.

Some other times when anti-depressants may be used

Other than postnatal depression, anti-depressants are also **sometimes** used to treat a variety of mental and physical health problems. These can include:

- Anxiety and tension.
- Panic attacks.
- Physical symptoms such as chronic (long-term) fatigue and pain.
- Obsessive-compulsive disorder (OCD).

Key point

It's important to ask your doctor the reason why you may be prescribed an anti-depressant.

Frequently asked questions

Q Why do doctors use anti-depressant medication for treating depression?

Remember the Five Areas model: there are links between the changes that happen in your thinking, your feelings, your behaviour and your body if you have depression. Because of the links between each of the areas, the **physical treatment** offered by medication can lead to improvements in the other areas too.

Five Areas assessment

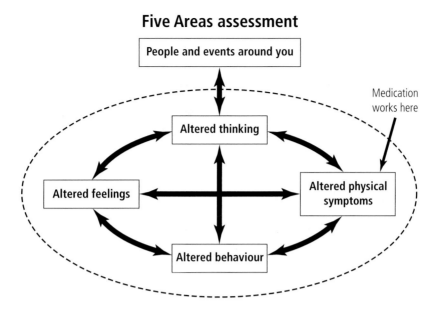

Q How well do anti-depressant tablets work?

About two-thirds of mothers who have severe or moderate postnatal depression find that taking anti-depressants helps lift their symptoms. Many people believe they get the best out of them when you're also having a talking treatment such as cognitive behaviour therapy (CBT) or interpersonal psychotherapy (IPT) at the same time, however they can also be used alone.

Q How long do they take to work?

Don't expect immediate results. Anti-depressant medicines take about two to four weeks to begin to work. And it may take up to four to six weeks for their positive effects to show.

Therefore it's very important that you take the tablets regularly and for long enough, even if to begin with they seem like they aren't working. Sometimes, doctors tell you to take a smaller dose of the anti-depressant medicine to start with. Then they may slowly increase the dose over several weeks/months if this is needed.

Key point

So you shouldn't give up on your anti-depressant medicine if you don't notice changes straight away.

Q Do anti-depressants have side effects?

All tablets have side effects. The important question is whether the side effects of having untreated depression are worse. The modern anti-depressant medicines that are used in postnatal depression usually have few side effects. For example, they usually don't cause much drowsiness.

Many side effects disappear within a few days of starting the tablets as you get used to them. Sometimes anxiety can actually worsen how much we notice our symptoms. Your doctor should have gone through the possible side effects with you when you started treatment. But you can always ask them again if you are unsure. You can also read the patient information leaflet that comes with the tablets.

Q Can I drive or use machinery if I take tablets?

Many anti-depressant medications can affect your ability to drive and operate machinery. They can also increase the effects of alcohol. Read the patient information leaflet that you would have received with your prescription to see if this applies to you. Or ask your doctor if you have any doubts.

Q What if I might be pregnant again?

If you're pregnant you may worry about taking medications. If you are already on medication then you shouldn't suddenly stop taking it. It's important that you discuss with your doctor or other health professional you are in contact with about what you should do.

So if you think you may be pregnant, **tell your doctor straight away**. Sometimes your doctor may suggest starting anti-depressants during pregnancy. You and your doctor will balance the pros and cons of taking tablets for you and your unborn baby. Remember it's also important for your baby that you are getting the most appropriate treatment for your depression.

Q Can I breastfeed and also take an anti-depressant?

If you are breastfeeding, some of the medication may pass in the milk to your baby. It's usually possible for your doctor to choose an anti-depressant that is less likely to cause problems for your baby.

Your attitudes towards medication

I worry that they are addictive

Anti-depressants are **not** addictive in the way that some other drugs are, but **stopping them in one go may cause you to have unpleasant withdrawal effects**. You don't get addicted to modern anti-depressants in the same way as you can to alcohol or tablets such as benzodiazepines (see below).

If you start by taking the tablets at too high a dose, you are more likely to get side effects. To prevent this, your doctor may suggest you start by taking a small dose of your medication and then increasing the dose. In the same way, when you are ready to stop taking the tablets, your doctor will taper down the dose over several weeks or months. That means your doctor and you must together make a careful timetable for reducing your medication. **Don't consider stopping your medication on your own**.

I think I should get better on my own without taking tablets

Taking anti-depressant medications is one of many important ways of helping yourself to get better. They can helpfully change some of the physical symptoms that you get in depression. They also boost how you feel. They don't replace the need for you to work at changing other things in your life, such as tackling relationship problems or other practical problems. It's important when you have a young baby to try to get better as quickly as possible. Many anti-depressants begin to show benefits within only a few weeks. If you are in any doubt, discuss this with your doctor.

Key point

Remember, our body, thoughts and feelings are all part of us – they are not in separate boxes. If you break your leg, you are unlikely to say 'I want to get better by myself without medical treatment'. So why do this if you're having depression? If your doctor recommends that you take anti-depressants, discuss why they are suggesting this. You should jointly make the decision about whether it's the right thing for you at the moment.

My family and friends are unhappy I'm taking tablets

Sometimes people can have strong views about anti-depressant tablets. As in the example above about the broken leg, the best advice they could offer is that if your doctor suggests a treatment that's known to work well, you should try it.

This won't always mean taking tablets, although tablets can often be an important part of your overall treatment package. Your family should know that your doctor will have taken into account that you are pregnant or breastfeeding.

Practical problems you may have while taking medication

Remembering to take your tablets

For almost any medication, it may be hard to remember to take them on a regular basis. You might want to try:

- Getting into a routine. Take the tablets at a set time each day.

- Placing the tablets somewhere where you will see them when you need to take them. For example, placing them by your toothbrush.

- Writing little notes to yourself saying **Medication**.

- Using coloured pieces of paper to help remind you if you don't want other people to read your notes.

- Put the date when to request a further repeat prescription in your diary so you have at least three days before your tablets run out.

- Setting an alarm in your watch, an alarm clock or using the alarm function on a mobile phone to remind you to take them at a set time.

- Asking other people to remind you/phone you if you find that you struggle to remember otherwise. If you feel this way, your doctor may suggest that someone else keep them for you.

- **Please note**: tablets can be dangerous if taken in overdose or by someone they aren't prescribed for. Ensure young children don't take any tablets by mistake.

I sometimes take a higher dose than is prescribed

You should never do this. It can be tempting to take extra tablets at times of higher distress to cope, even when your doctor hasn't prescribed the medicine with this in mind. It may be **dangerous**, and most likely it won't help in any way. This is because of the particular way in which anti-depressants work. It means they will not help you feel better at the time you take the higher dose anyway.

Key point

Remember: taking more tablets than your doctor has told you to take can backfire and worsen how you feel. This is because taking tablets at higher than recommended doses may cause you to have unpleasant side effects. It may be **dangerous** because it wrongly teaches you that you're only managing to cope because of using the medication. You then may come to believe that you can't live life without the tablets.

Stopping anti-depressants

Sometimes people can be tempted to stop taking medication without telling their doctor. You may be afraid you are letting them down, or that you will be 'told off' if you do. But it's actually better to discuss any worries you have openly with your doctor. It's also important when stopping anti-depressants to do this gradually, by making a timetable with your doctor. Otherwise, you may get withdrawal symptoms.

Key point

Stopping an anti-depressant too early is the commonest cause of worsening depression. The national guidelines advise doctors to tell their patients to continue to take the anti-depressant medication for at least six months after feeling better to prevent slipping back into depression. If you have had several bouts of depression your doctor may recommend you take tablets for at least two years after feeling better.

Putting things into practice

If you want to find out more about the use of anti-depressant medications please discuss this with your doctor. They will be able to suggest other sources of information about the treatments that are available.

Summary

In this workbook you have learnt:

- How anti-depressants are used.
- The answer to some common questions about anti-depressants.
- Some useful hints and tips to get the best out of medication.
- The pros and cons of medication if this is being suggested for you.

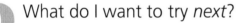 What have I learnt from this workbook?

What do I want to try *next*?

My notes

Overcoming Postnatal Depression
A Five Areas Approach

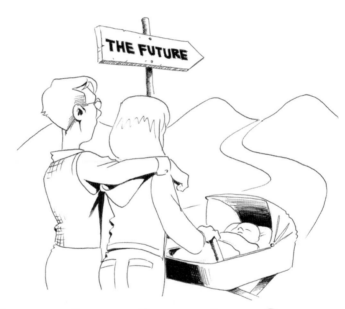

Planning for the future

www.livinglifetothefull.com
www.fiveareas.com

Dr Chris Williams, Dr Roch Cantwell and
Karen Robertson

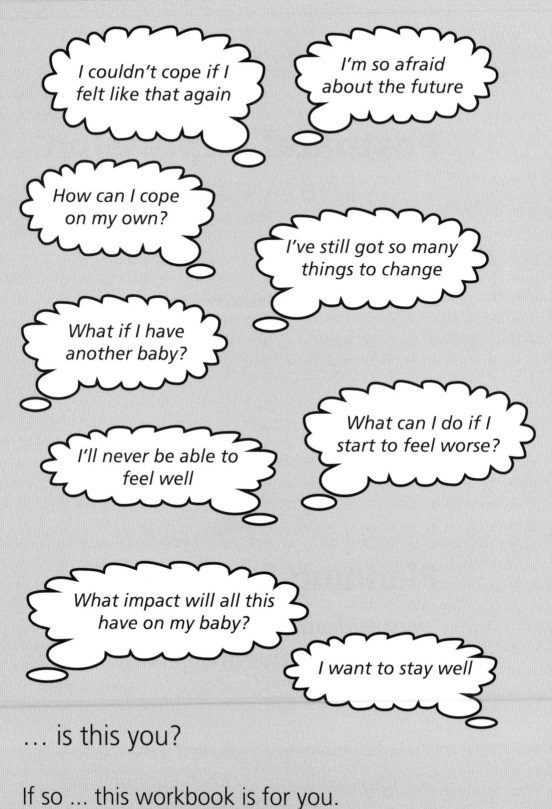

... is this you?

If so ... this workbook is for you.

In this workbook you will:

- Look back at what you have learned in this course.

- Summarise key lessons you have learned.

- Work out 'danger signs' that will alert you that things may be slipping back.

- Make a clear plan to stay well.

- Set up some **Review days** so **you** can check your own progress.

The journey of recovery

It can sometimes be helpful to think of yourself as being on a **journey of recovery**. When you first started this course, you probably had lots of different problems you wished to tackle.

By using the course workbooks we hope things have improved in at least some areas since you began your journey down this path. In the following sections there are some questions to help you identify **what has been helpful for you** to move on.

My journey

 Task

Q What is different now from before?

Q What gains have I made?

Q How have things changed/improved in each of the five areas?

Area 1a:
How have things changed/improved in the situations, and practical problems I face?

Area 1b:
What practical resources have I discovered in myself and in the support from others around me? (For example, how to build close relationships.)

Area 2:
How have things changed/improved in my thinking?

Areas 3 and 4:
How have things changed/improved in my feelings and the physical symptoms I used to have? (For example, you may still have the same worries and fears, but not believe them as much, or be troubled by them as often.)

Area 5:

How have things changed/improved in my behaviour and activity levels? What can I do now and what can't I still do? Do I respond to things in helpful or unhelpful ways? (For example, have you been more active, faced your fears and done things that give you a sense of pleasure and made you feel close to other people.)

Working out what's made the difference

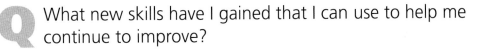 What have I done to make these changes happen?

What new skills have I gained that I can use to help me continue to improve?

How can I continue to use what I have learned in my everyday life?

Q What things might get in the way of me doing this?

(For example, my baby's needs, other family members or parents not getting on, major commitments or interruptions to my usual routine.)

What practical steps can I take to continue making changes?

Some things to do

> **Example: Sally's mental fitness plan**
>
> - When I begin to feel low and stressed, I need to do something about it before it worsens.
> - Don't withdraw from others when I feel down – they can really help me pick up.
> - When I feel overwhelmed by problems – just tackle them one at a time.

📌 Task

Now answer the questions below to help make your own plan.

Some things to do	Tick here if this affects your life – even if just sometimes
Tackle things early if you feel worse	☐
Build on your strengths/resources	☐
Stop, think and reflect on negative thoughts	☐
Don't let extreme and unhelpful thinking take over	☐
Keep doing things that you value (that is, those activities that give you a sense of pleasure, achievement and closeness to other people)	☐
Face up to your fears – don't let avoidance take over	☐
Live reasonably healthily – being active, eating, sleeping – but not obsessively so	☐
Say no – balance demands you put on yourself	☐
Allow space and time for you	☐
Use relaxation tapes or techniques if you find them helpful, such as the Anxiety Control Training technique described on the Living Life to the Full website (**www.livinglifetothefull.com**). This can be downloaded from **www.fiveareas.com**	☐
If you are prescribed an anti-depressant medication, take it regularly. Discuss any changes you want to make with your own doctor	☐

Some things *not* to do	Tick here if this affects your life – even if just sometimes
Letting problems build up and not dealing with them	☐
Letting your thinking spiral out of control	☐
Avoiding things or putting things off	☐
Doing things that end up backfiring/worsening things (for example, taking on too much or setting yourself up to fail)	☐
Drinking too much or even blocking how you feel using street drugs	☐

Q What else have I learned about getting and staying better?

Staying well: watching out for the problem times

One important thing to do now is watch out for your problem times. If you do this, you can plan in advance what you're going to do if you start to feel worse for whatever reason. This could happen when you experience some:

● Personal loss: when you feel let down, rejected or abandoned by someone, for example, lose a friendship or suffer a bereavement.

● Setbacks or challenges – for example personal or family illness or unemployment.

● Stress: when you think things are beginning to get out of control. For example, it's common for mothers to find it stressful for a time when they first return to work after having a baby.

Key point

The key is not to think that you need to avoid these problem times.
Instead the challenge is to find ways of tackling them that will help sort
out your problem.

Q In which situations am I likely to suffer setbacks?

Q What do I need to do differently if I encounter these
situations?

**Example: Julia identifies her early warning
signs**

- **People and events**: Feeling overwhelmed by problems and not acting to
  overcome them.
- **Altered thinking**: Becoming very negative and predicting that things will go
  badly (negative predictions). Having a very negative view of myself. Overlooking
  good things that happen (negative mental filter). Worrying too much about my
  baby's health (catastrophising).
- **Altered feelings**: Feeling low and weepy, and also feeling very little at all, as
  though my feelings are becoming numb.
- **Altered physical feelings/symptoms**: Feeling very low in energy and
  finding it hard to get up in the morning. Noticing my sleep pattern worsening.

- **Altered behaviour**: A tendency to want to withdraw and ask my sister not to visit. Stopping doing things I normally enjoy, such as going for a walk or going to the shops. Starting to snack more when I feel stressed.

Julia identifies one key early warning sign:

I am going to watch out for times when I start to avoid people by staying in and not answering the phone.

This key early warning sign means: Do something now to tackle how you feel.

Your early warning signs

Task

Now make your list of early warning signs.

People and events around you (Area 1)

Altered thinking (Area 2)

Altered feelings/emotions (Area 3)

Altered physical symptoms (Area 4)

Altered behaviour/activity levels (Area 5)

My **key** early warning sign(s)

Making an emergency plan

Imagine one day you hear a smoke alarm bleeping while you're watching TV. What do you do? **Do you ignore it** and keep watching TV as if there was no problem? Or do you get up to find out if there is a problem, and, if there is, try to deal with it?

Key point

You need to have planned what you do in response to your key early warning sign(s).

Try to think of other people while making your plan:

- **Respond helpfully**. Keep doing your activities, things that give you pleasure and a sense of achievement. Maintain your healthy helpful habits. Do what has helped you before.

- **Choose to stay in contact with people who support you**. Choose not to isolate yourself – tell others you trust that you are noticing some problems.

- **Talk to a healthcare practitioner** about your problems and discuss whether you need more help. You may talk to someone you know about how you feel, or your health visitor, or your doctor may refer you to a mental health specialist such as a clinical psychologist, psychiatrist or nurse.

An **emergency plan** can help you to tackle any early warning signs you notice.

The following example shows how Julia decides to react to her early warning signs.

Example: Julia's early warning sign emergency plan

My planned response

Altered thinking: with negative predictions and mind-reading	I need to identify and challenge extreme and unhelpful thinking
Altered feelings: feeling low and weepy	Do the above things, and also go to see my health visitor or doctor to talk about whether other help or support may be useful
Altered physical symptoms: feeling low in energy, and worse in the morning	Plan to do more difficult tasks later on in the day. Do things at a reasonable pace
Altered behaviour: withdrawing from doing things I like	Create an action plan to do things that give me a sense of pleasure, achievement, or closeness to others
Altered behaviour: asking my friends not to visit	Choose to ask people over each week for a short period of time

Your emergency response plan

Q What is your **emergency plan** in case you have a setback?

Try to be very clear about the things you could do. Include your own mental fitness plan as well as any people you could contact to ask for help. Going back to the example of the smoke alarm on page 371 – if a fire was beginning to worsen at home in spite of your attempts to tackle it, you would call for professional help. Similarly, if you feel worse in spite of your emergency plan, you should get in touch with someone who can help. They can advise you whether other approaches may be helpful.

How to plan a regular review day

Mark the last day of each month on your calendar as a 'review' day. During this review time, try to spend 30 minutes or so thinking back over the previous month. You can plan to do the review day more often if you wish (for example, every two weeks).

Key point

The important thing is trying to commit yourself to do your review regularly over the long term.

Here are some ideas about how to go about your review.

My review day:

Date:

Since my last review:

What's gone well?

What hasn't gone so well?

Am I slipping back? (review your warning signs list or emergency plan if needed)

What can I learn from what has happened?

How can I put what has been learned into practice?

My plan for the next few weeks (consider short, medium and long-term changes):

What am I going to do?

When am I going to do it?

What can prevent this happening? (What problems could arise, and how can I overcome these? What might not let me put my plan into action)

How will I try to make sure that I carry out my plan?

Date of my next review (Do I need to do this more often?):

Summary

In this workbook you have:

- Looked back at what you have learned.

- Identified the key lessons you have learned.

- Learnt about your 'danger signs' that tell you things may be slipping back.

- Learnt how to make a clear plan to stay well.

- Set up some review days so **you can check** your progress.

 What have I learnt from this workbook?

 What do I want to try *next*?

Sources of extra help

- **Your family doctor or GP**. Your GP can offer medical advice and (if they feel it is necessary) refer you to a mental health specialist for a detailed assessment.

- **Social services**. Social services can be a great source of support for families. You can find your local social services office hours' enquiry phone number and a 24-hour emergency phone number in the *Yellow Pages*.

Other organisations you can approach are:

- Local counselling services, such as **Relate**, which helps people having relationship difficulties (see **www.relate.org.uk**).

- **The Royal College of Psychiatrists** – the college has factsheets about postnatal depression and more (see **www.rcpsych.ac.uk**).

You can buy the following helpful books from local or online bookshops including **www.fiveareas.com/books** or you may find them at your local library:

- *Overcoming Anxiety: A Five Areas Approach* by Chris Williams

- *Overcoming Depression and Low Mood: A Five Areas Approach* by Chris Williams

- *I'm Not Supposed to Feel Like This: A Christian Self-help Approach to Depression and Anxiety* by Chris Williams, Paul Richards and Ingrid Whitton

- *Overcoming Low Self-Esteem: A Self-Help Guide to Using Cognitive Behavioural Techniques* by Melanie Fennell

- *Mind Over Mood* by Christine Padesky and Dennis Greenberger

 www.livinglifetothefull.com

This website has free online training courses that teach key life skills by using the same model used in this book. There are useful additional handouts as well as DVD-based videos to learn key life skills confidentially and for free.

The main Five Areas resource site is **www.fiveareas.com**

A request for feedback

Finally, you have now finished this course. Well done! We hope it has been helpful. The content of the Five Areas courses is updated and improved on a regular basis. This is based on feedback from users and practitioners. If there are areas in the workbooks that you found hard to understand, or that seemed unclear, please let us know. However, please note that we cannot provide any specific advice on treatment.

To provide feedback please contact us:

Via email: **feedback@fiveareas.com**

Or you can write to us at:

Five Areas, PO Box 9, Glasgow G63 0WL

In your feedback, please state which workbook or book you are referring to.

My notes